Intermittent Fasting For Women After 50

Learn to Make 200 Delicious Recipes and Take Control of Your Health with Intermittent Fasting

MICHELLE GLISSON

Table of Contents

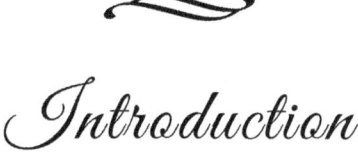

Introduction

Aging is a natural process, and everyone must go through it. The process accelerates in women when they hit 50 because of natural hormonal changes and pre-menopausal symptoms. This is the time that women should take extra care of their health and well-being. It would help if you took into considerations all the aspects of your body and health. At 50, your bone density starts lowering at a regular pace, the calcium gets depleted, and you will be prone to heart and neurological disease. All this information is not to scare you but to explain things in matter of fact without sugar-coating anything.

This book is specifically designed for women entering their fifties and is concerned about their health and well-being. In this book, we introduce Intermittent Fasting. This is an eating routine that you can develop as a lifestyle. Theis lifestyle has numerous advantages such as:

- Lower risk of heart disease

- Lower risk of neurological disorders

- Insulin levels become balanced and prevent diabetes.

- Weight loss

- Muscle gain

- Body detoxification

So, what is this magic technique to achieve so much? You must make few changes to your daily eating habits, and you will well be on your journey to your best health.

Intermittent fasting is a system in which you fast for a specific period, and then you have an eating window in which you can consume food. The best part about this way of fasting is that none of the food groups are off-limits. We should consider that, though no food groups are restricted, we should be thoughtful of what we put in our bodies. The food we consume should be healthy and can impart energy for longer periods. When we look at macro food groups, we see that carbohydrates give us instant energy and are utilized quickly. However, in proteins and fats, the energy is released slowly and spread over a long time. So, it is advisable to consume these macromolecules while intermittent fasting. Another benefit of consuming more protein and fat is that they do not give you an instant sugar spike. In this book, you will find recipes that are suitable for you when following intermittent fasting.

The different types of intermittent fasting commonly followed are:

1. 16:8 fasting.

2. 20:4 fasting, also known as Warrior Fasting.

3. 24-hour fasting on alternate days.

4. 5:2 fasting.

Chapter 1.

Basics of Intermittent Fasting

You may have come across the term intermittent fasting. Intermittent fasting is a diet where you fast for regular intervals for short or long periods. However, consumption of non-caloric beverages is permitted during the fast. This method of eating is adapted mostly for weight loss, but it has many other health benefits. The health benefits include:

- Low insulin levels
- Fat burn due to release of noradrenaline
- Prevention of heart disease
- Prevention of neurological disorders
- Prevention of diabetes
- Weight loss

Taking care of your health habits is important throughout your life, but it becomes more important when you reach a certain age. A person should be more careful regarding health and well-being decisions when they are reaching their fifties. This is because the metabolic rates slow down, and calcium depletion rapidly occurs, especially in women. Another reason why women should be more concerned about their health in their fifties because of the onset of menopause. This is a phase where the aging process is accelerated, and if you do not take care of your body, your systems become weaker. Therefore, women should be more concerned about taking control of their health and well-being when nearing their fifties.

Intermittent fasting is an excellent option for women. It is easy to follow, and the best part is that intermittent fasting does not restrict any food groups, unlike other diets.

1.1. How Does it Work?

When you eat, your body produces a chemical called insulin, which breaks down carbohydrates into smaller molecules for consumption. But when you fast, your insulin levels go down, and your fat deposits are prompted to release energy for consumption. This way you lose weight. Lower insulin levels are also essential to prevent diabetes.

Another hormone known as noradrenaline is activated while fasting. This hormone prompts the fat cells to release energy in the absence of other available calories. All this causes your fat deposits to decrease.

1.2. Types of Intermittent Fasting

There are several types of methods to follow when you are intermittent fasting. Following are the common types of intermittent fasting:

- 16:8 fasting.

This method is by far the most popular method of fasting. It is the easiest to follow. In this method, you follow the fasting routine every day for 16 hours, and you have an 8-hour eating window. When you are in the fasting phase, you should consume non-caloric beverages.

- 5:2 fasting.

This is also a popular method of intermittent fasting. In this method, you fast for two days a week. During the whole fasting day, you are only allowed to consume ¼ of your normal intake. If you consume 2000 calories daily, you will only consume 500 calories on a fast day.

- Warrior Fasting

This is almost the same as the 16:8 fast, but the only difference is that it is 20:4 fast. You have an eating window of only 4 hours and a fasting period of 20 hours in this fast. This is a rather extreme method of intermittent fasting.

- Alternate Day Fast

In this style of fasting, you fast every other day. One day you eat normally, and the other day you fast. During the 24 hours fast, you can only consume up to 500 calories if your normal intake is 2000 calories.

1.3. The Best for You

Now that you have a basic understanding of the most common intermittent fasting practices. If you consider the practicality, the two most suitable types for you will be:

- 16:8 fasting.

- 5:2 fasting.

These are simple and easy to follow and would not have any drastic effects on the body.

Chapter 2

Breakfast Recipes

We have always heard that breakfast is the most important meal of the day and we should consume breakfast first thing in the morning. But the latest research shows that this is not entirely necessary. All you must do is train your body correctly. You cannot deny the importance of the first meal of the day. About intermittent fasting, we will see breakfast recipes as the first meal to break your fast. The following chapter has a variety of recipes that you can kick-start your day with.

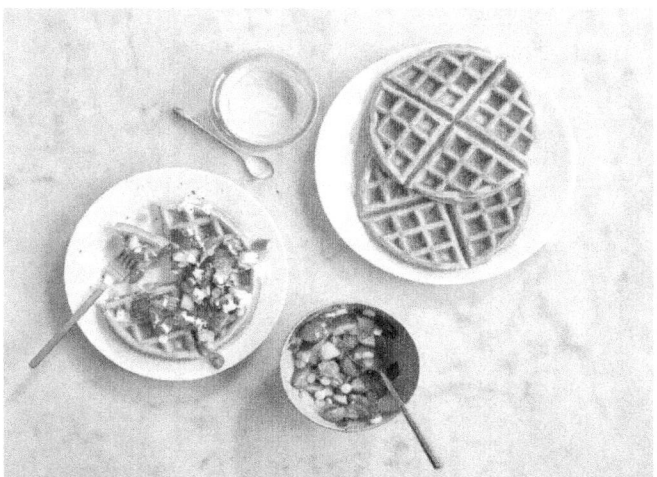

2.1. Oats with roasted veggies

This recipe is energy-packed and full of protein and vitamins. This is a perfect recipe to start your eating window.

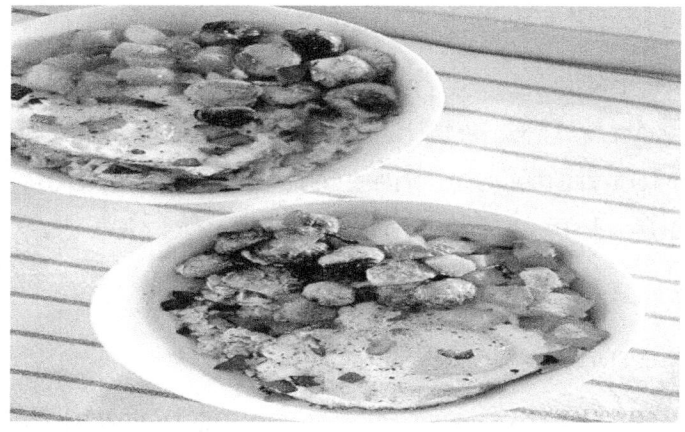

- Total Time: 30 minutes

- Prep. Time: 10 minutes

- Cooking Time: 20 minutes

- Serving Size: 2 servings

Ingredients:

1. 1 cup Brussel sprouts (halved)

2. 2 cups butternut squash (cubed)

3. 1 big onion (chopped)

4. 2 tbsp olive oil

5. 1 tsp black pepper

6. 1 tsp salt

7. 1 tbsp butter

8. 1 cup old-fashioned oats

9. 2.5 cup water

10. 2 eggs

Instructions:

- Preheat an oven to 400∘F.

- Line a baking tray with butter paper and spread the Brussel sprouts, squash cubes and onions on the tray and sprinkle half tsp salt and half ½ tsp pepper.

- Bake for about 10 to 15 minutes till the vegetables are cooked.

- In a separate medium-sized pot, melt butter and roast the oats for 15 to 30 seconds. Add water and bring to boil. Add half tsp salt and half tsp pepper. Lower the flame and cook for 5 to 10 minutes until the oats' consistency gets thick but still liquid. Add more water if required. Take off from the heal and put it aside.

- Take out the vegetables from the oven.

- Fry two eggs with a sunny side up.

- For the presentation, take two cereal bowls and half of the oats to each bowl. Top it with a generous layer of vegetables.

- Next, top it with the egg.

- Enjoy your energy-packed breakfast.

2.2. Scrambled Eggs

This is one of the easiest breakfasts and quick to make. However, this recipe adds a healthier twist to an already healthy breakfast. This will keep your stomach full for a longer period. This recipe makes it easy for you to follow the intermittent lifestyle because it keeps your stomach filled for longer, and in turn, you consume lesser calories.

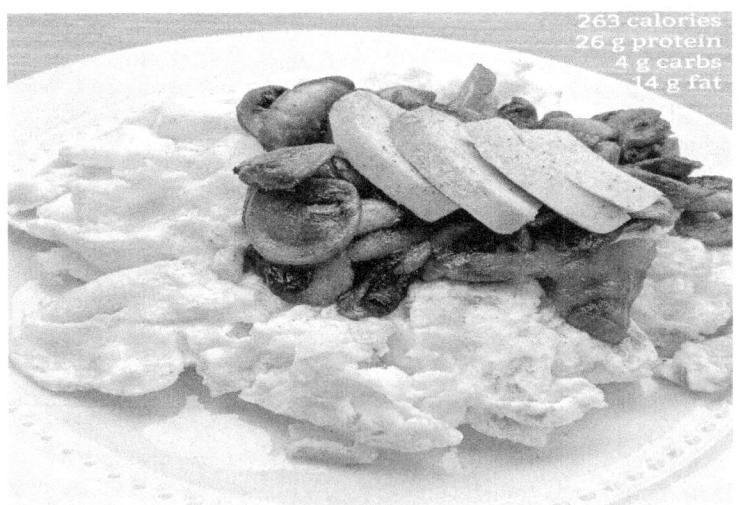

263 calories
26 g protein
4 g carbs
14 g fat

- Total Time: 10 mins

- Prep. Time: 5 mins

- Cooking Time: 5 mins

- Serving Size: 1-2 servings

Ingredients:

1. 1 medium egg
2. 2 egg whites
3. ½ cup mushroom
4. ½ ripe avocado sliced.
5. 2 tbsp olive oil

Instructions:

- In a skillet, put one 1 tbsp olive oil and put on the flame at medium. Add the egg whites and cook for 30 seconds, then add the full egg and keep on cooking. With a whisker, whisk the egg till it becomes firm. Take it out on a plate.

- Clean the skillet and add 1 tbsp olive oil.

- Sauté the mushroom for 2 minutes. Take care that they do not burn.

- Top the eggs with the cooked mushrooms and sliced avocado.

- Enjoy your meal.

2.3. Bulletproof Coffee

The bulletproof coffee is just a drink, but it helps you kickstart the day with ample energy that keeps you energized for a longer time. This can be used at the starting of the eating window and even end the eating window to keep you energized throughout the fast.

Total Time: 5 to mins

Prep. Time: 2 mins

Cook time: 2 mins.

Serving Size: 1 serving

Ingredients:

1. 2 tsp regular coffee
2. 1 ½ cup boiling water.
3. 1 tsp unsalted butter

4. 1 tsp coconut oil

Instructions:

- In a mug, prepare coffee by mixing the coffee with boiling water.

- Put this in a blender, add the butter and coconut oil.

- Blend on slow speed for 30 seconds and increase the speed.

- Blend for 1 more minute.

- Pour in a mug and enjoy your bullet of energy.

2.4. Avocado Toast

This is an easy and quick recipe that is packed with protein and healthy fat. It gives you an energy boost. It is best to use ripe avocadoes for this recipe. Underdone avocadoes may taste bitter and bland.

- Total Time: 15 mins

- Preparation Time: 10 mins

- Cooking Time: 5 minutes

- Serving Size: 1-2 servings

Ingredients:

1. 1 egg

2. 1 ripe avocado

3. 1 small onion is finely chopped.

4. 2 brown bread slices

5. ½ tsp salt

6. ½ tsp black pepper

Instructions:

- Hard boil the egg.

- Mash the avocado pulp in a medium-sized bowl.

- Mix the salt, pepper, and onion.

- When the egg is hard-boiled, peel it and mash it. Add it to the avocado mixture.

- Make the mixture smooth.

- Toast the bread slices.

- Spread the avocado spread on the toasted slices and enjoy.

2.5. Peach Smoothie

This is a fresh, fruity recipe that gives you a dose of vitamins to kick start your day. The recipe has a high amount of calcium which is good for your bone strength.

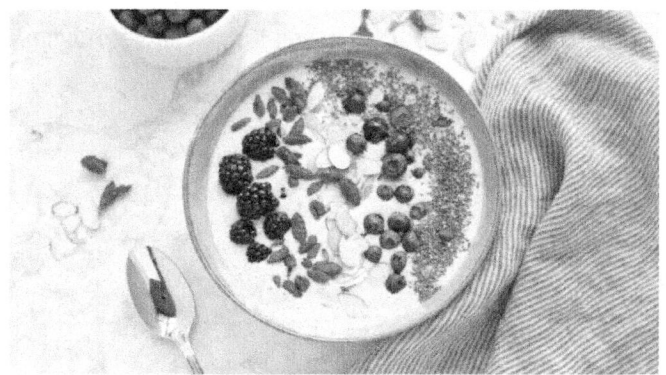

- Total Time: 15 mins

- Prep. Time: 15 mins

- Cooking Time: N/A

- Servings: 1 serving

Ingredients:

1. ½ cup yogurt

2. ½ cup coconut milk

3. 1 cup frozen peaches

4. ½ tsp chia seeds

5. Few blueberries

6. Silvered almonds for topping

Instructions:

- In a blender, add the peaches, coconut milk and yogurt.
- Blend the ingredients to make a smooth mixture.
- Pour it in a large glass or a cereal bowl.
- Top it with blueberries, chia seeds and almonds.
- Enjoy your smoothie.

2.6. Soymilk Oats Bowl

This recipe is for those people who avoid dairy or have some health restrictions for dairy. These oats bowl will provide you with all the essential food groups and makes a wonderful breakfast choice.

- Total Time: 15 mins
- Prep. Time: 5 mins
- Cooking Time: 10 minutes
- Serving Size: 1-2 servings

Ingredients:

1. 1 ½ cup soy milk
2. 2 tbsp steel cut oats
3. ½ tsp chia seeds (or powder)
4. ½ tsp flax seeds (or powder)
5. 1 tsp honey
6. 1 tsp dried raisins

Instructions:

- In a medium saucepan, add the soymilk and steel-cut oats.
- Cook for 10 minutes on a medium flame.
- See if the oats are cooked and pour them into the cereal bowl.

- Top with all the remaining ingredients.

- Enjoy your healthy bowl.

2.7. Almond Granola

Granola is your savior on those early mornings when you are in a rush. A good thing about granola is that you can grab and go. This recipe makes granola about 8 to 10 servings and can last for over a month in an air-tight container.

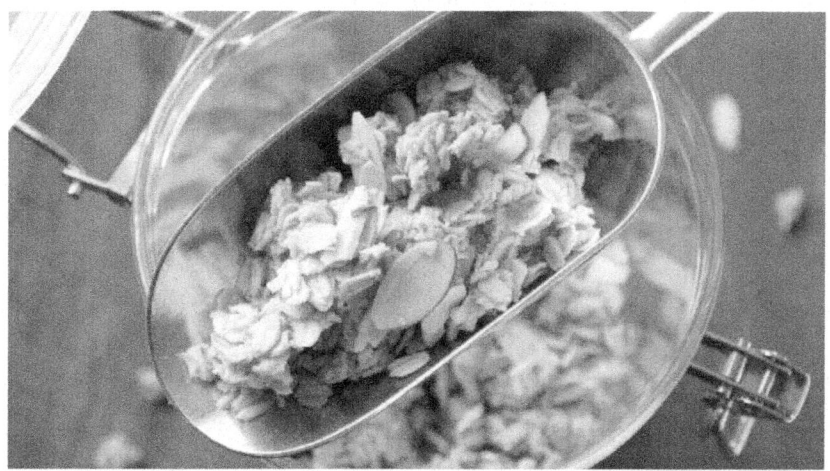

- Total Time: 2 hours 10 minutes

- Prep. Time: 10 minutes

- Cooking Time: 2 hours

- Serving Size: 8-10 servings

Ingredients:

1. 3 cups old-fashioned oats

2. ¾ cup slivered almonds

3. 1 tsp salt

4. ½ cup sugar

5. 1 tsp vanilla extract

6. ½ cup water

7. ½ cup grapeseed oil

Instructions:

- Preheat the oven to 200°F.

- Prepare a cookie sheet by lining it with butter paper.

- In a bowl, mix the oats and almonds.

- In a saucepan, mix the sugar and salt. Add water and heat it on a medium flame.

- Add the vanilla extract. When the salt and sugar are mixed, add the grapeseed oil.

- Stir it and add it to the oats and almond mixture.

- Mix the sugar syrup to the oats. Spread this mixture on the baking tray.

- Bake for two hours and take out of the oven.

- Store in an air-tight container for up to a month.

2.8. Mushroom Omelet

Eggs are a staple for breakfast and are highly encouraged when following an intermittent fasting routine. Sometimes we feel that plain eggs get boring. For times like those, this recipe is perfect. With the right amount of protein and vitamins, this is your best choice for a healthy breakfast.

- Total Time: 10 mins

- Prep. Time: 5 mins

- Cook Time: 5mins

- Serving: 1-2 servings

Ingredients:

1. 3 eggs

2. ½ cup sliced mushroom

3. 1 small onion finely chipped

4. ¼ tsp salt

5. ¼ tsp pepper

6. 2 tbsp olive oil

Instructions:

- Break three eggs in a medium-size mixing bowl.

- Add the sliced mushrooms, salt, pepper, and onions.

- Mix well.

- In a frying pan, pour the oil and heat on medium flame.

- Pour half of the egg batter into the pan and let it cook for 1 minute.

- Then very carefully turn over the egg and cook on the other side for 1 minute.

- Take out the omelet on a plate.

- Repeat the same procedure with the remaining egg batter.

- Enjoy the eggs with bread or eat separately.

2.9. Egg Salad

This is a simple egg salad recipe. You can eat it as it is or spread it on bread. Both ways, this is a delicious variation you can try for breakfast.

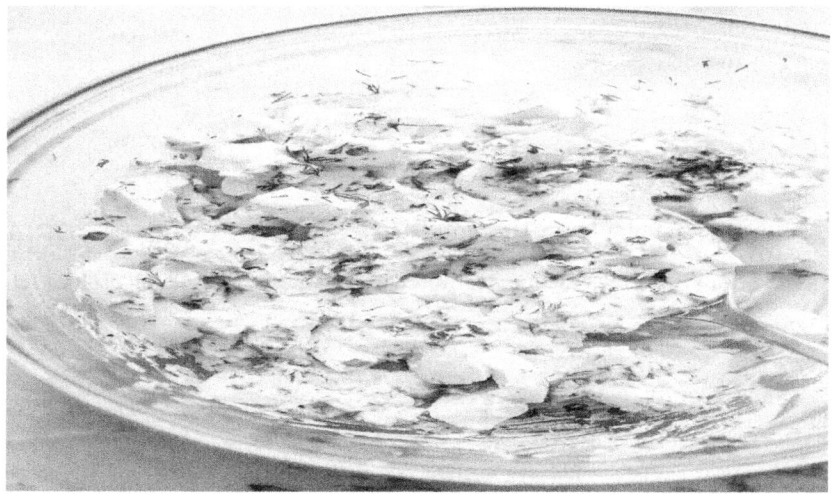

- Total Time: 20 mins

- Prep. Time: 5 mins

- Cook Time: 15 mins

- Serving Size: 1-2 servings

Ingredients:

1. 3 large eggs
2. 2 tsp dill (chopped)
3. 1 tsp chives (minced)
4. 1 tsp mustard
5. ¼ tsp salt
6. 2 tsp mayonnaise
7. ¼ tsp black pepper

Instructions:

- Hard boil the three eggs and bring them to cool.

- When the eggs are at room temperature, peel them and cut them into small pieces.

- Put the eggs in a bowl and mix all the remaining ingredients lightly such that the eggs still retain the shape. Eggs should not be mashed.

- The salad is ready. Consume it as it is or spread it on bread and enjoy the egg salad sandwich.

2.10. Poached Egg and Toast

This recipe is delicious and simple to prepare. When you are intermittent fasting, you always must take care that all you eat has beneficial nutritional value. This helps the body keep working efficiently when you are in your fasting state.

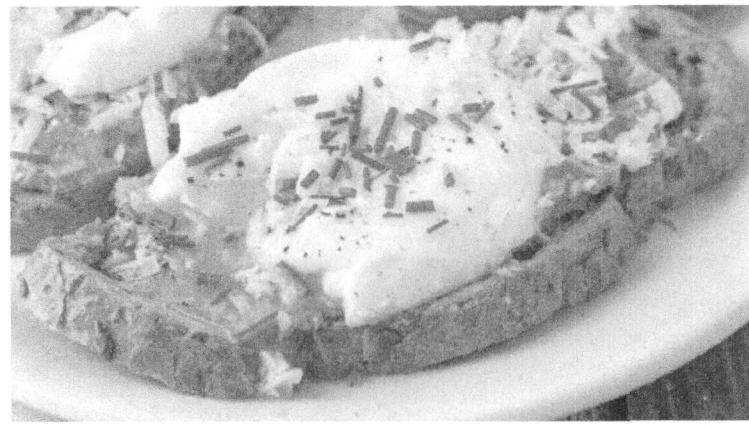

- Total Time: 10 mins

- Prep. Time: 5 mins

- Cooking Time: 5 mins

- Serving Size: 1-2 servings

Ingredients:

1. 2 large eggs

2. 1 large avocado

3. 2 tsp lemon juice

4. 2 brown bread slices

5. 50 g butter

6. ¼ /tsp salt

7. ¼ tsp pepper

8. 50 g grated cheese to top

9. 1 tsp chives to garnish

Instructions:

- Cut the avocado and take out the flesh. Mash it in a bowl with a fork. Add lemon juice, salt, and pepper. Mix and prepare a smooth mixture.

- Toast the bread slices.

- Spread the toasts with a layer of butter, then a layer of avocado spread.

- Poach the two eggs and put the mon top of the bread slices.

- Top the eggs with cheese and chives.

2.11. Perfect Hard-Boiled Eggs

Eggs are a wonderful food for weight loss and muscle gain. There are many ways to hard-boil eggs, but this is one tried and tested recipe.

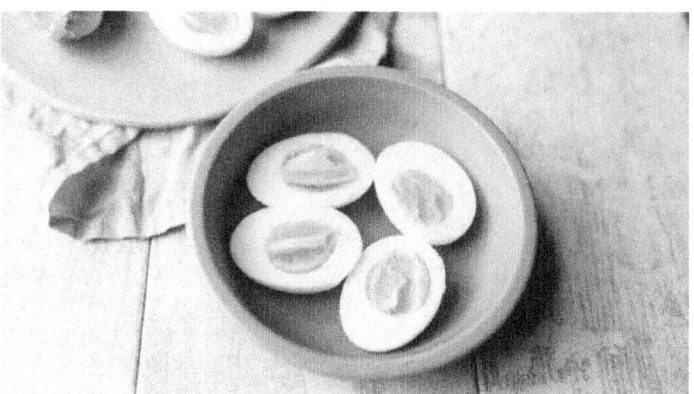

- Total Time: 25 mins
- Prep. Time: N/A
- Cooking Time: 5 mins
- Serving Size: 2 servings

Ingredients:

1. 4 eggs
2. 5 cups water.
3. Pinch of salt
4. Pinch of pepper

Instructions:

- In a medium saucepan, add the eggs and pour them over the water.
- Turn on the stove and bring the water to boil. Let it boil for 1 whole minute, and then remove the flame.
- Cover the saucepan and leave for 20 minutes.
- After 20 mins remove the water and wash the eggs under cold water and easily peel the eggs.
- Cut the eggs in half and garnish them with salt and pepper.

- When intermittent fasting, you must consume two hard-boiled eggs.

2.12. Overnight Oats

This is a simple and yummy recipe that you can prepare at night to have breakfast in the morning. It can be prepared in a bowl or a jar.

- Total Time: 10 mins
- Prep. Time: 5 mins
- Cooking Time: N/A
- Serving Size: 1 serving

Ingredients:

1. ½ cup yogurt
2. 2 tbsp oats
3. 1 tsp honey
4. 3 strawberries sliced.
5. ¼ cup milk
6. 1 tsp flax seeds
7. 4 blueberries
8. 1tsp chia seeds

Instructions:

- In a mason jar, add the oats, then top with milk.
- Next, add the yogurt and the remaining ingredients.
- Put the jar in the fridge and let it stay overnight.
- Enjoy this pudding in the morning.

2.13. Granola Bars

These granola bars can be prepared and kept in an airtight container for up to 2 months. These bars are good for people who are on the go most of the time, and intermittent fasting cannot be practiced easily.

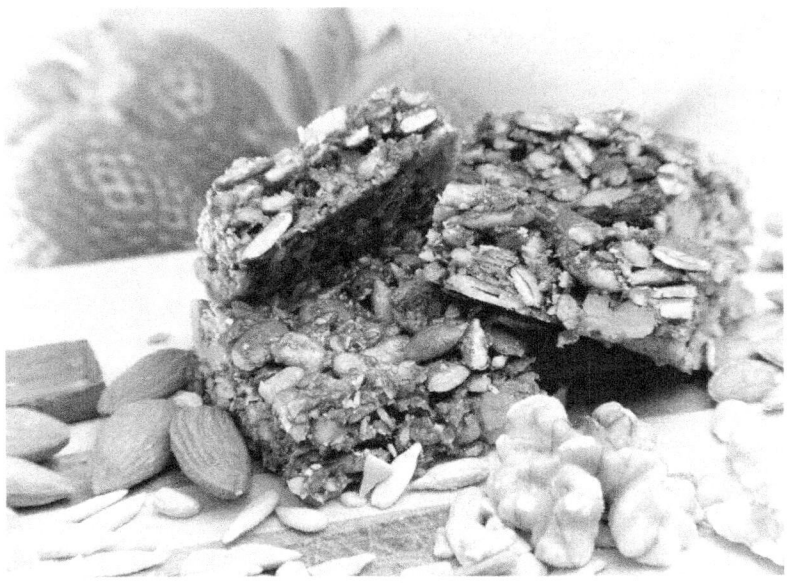

- Total Time: 1 hour 10 mins
- Prep Time: 30 mins
- Cooking Time: 40 mins
- Serving Size: 24 bars

Ingredients:

1. 1 cup almonds cut.
2. 1/2 cup of thinly cut dried apricots.
3. ¼ tsp salt
4. ½ cup walnuts cut.
5. ½ cup of wheat germ
6. 1 1/2 cup grated coconut.
7. 1/2 cup sunflower seeds
8. 1/4 cup golden raisins
9. 1/4 cup black raisins

10. 1 ½ cup honey

11. ½ cup pumpkin seeds

12. 7 tbsp brown sugar

13. 2 tsp vanilla essence

14. 6 tbsp soft butter

Instructions:

- Turn on the oven at 350 °F.

- Mix the oats, almonds, and all the other dried nuts you wish to use in a big bowl.

- Transfer this mixture into a cookie dish.

- Roast this mixture over a light flame for 10 minutes, sometimes stirring it till the mixture starts to brown.

- Put the mixture in the wide bowl again and add the wheat germ, pumpkin, and sunflower seeds.

- Switch the oven heat down to 280 °F.

- Stir together honey, butter, vanilla essence, brown sugar, and salt in a saucepan.

- Boil the mixture on low flame; let it simmer. Remove from the flame.

- Use a wooden spoon to fold in the dry ingredients.

- Finally, fold in the raisins and apricots to the mix.

- Prepare a cookie tray by greasing it with butter or cooking oil. Line it with butter paper.

- Press the granola into the tray so that it is spread evenly on the cookie tray. Bake this for about 20-30 minutes. See that the granola has achieved a light brown tinge.

- Take out from the oven. Let it cool. Use a knife to loosen the edges. Turn over the cookie tray on the counter. A slab of granola should be formed.

- Peel away the butter paper. Use a knife to cut it into smaller pieces.

- The bars have attained a shape but are still easily crumbled. So, it is better that after cooling, you wrap them in individual plastic sheets.

- If you want crunchy bars, follow the next step.

- Put the cut bars back to the cookie tray. And bake for 5 minutes.
- Let the bars cool. Wrap each bar in a separate plastic sheet.
- Keep in a cool and dry place.
- Store in an airtight container for up to a month.

2.14. Baked Beans with Veggies

This baked bean recipe is easy to make and is full of dietary fiber and essential vitamins.

- Total Time: 40 mins
- Prep Time: 10 mins
- Cooking Time: 30 mins
- Serving Size: 4 servings

Ingredients:

1. 2 cans baked beans.
2. 1 onion diced.
3. 2 tbsp olive oil
4. 1 tomato diced.
5. 1 carrot diced.
6. 1 tbsp sugar
7. 3 tbsp tomato ketchup
8. 1 tbsp vinegar
9. 2 tbsp Worcestershire sauce
10. 2 garlic cloves minced.
11. 2 celery sticks chopped.

Instructions:

- In a large saucepan, add the oil and onions. Stir fry for 3 minutes and add the garlic. Stir fry for one minute and add the carrots. Add ¼ cup of water and cook. When the water is dried, add the tomatoes and celery. Keep stirring, and then add the baked beans.

- Cook for 2 to 3 mins and then add salt, sugar, vinegar, Worcestershire sauce and ketchup.

- Cook for 5 more minutes and turn of the flame.

- Serve with scrambled eggs and baked mushrooms.

2.15. Sausage Muffins

This is a favorite recipe and easy to make. These are a perfect savory breakfast for you.

- Total Time: 30 mins

- Prep. Time: 10 mins

- Cooking Time: 20 mins

- Serving Size: 2-3 servings

Ingredients:

1. 2 eggs

2. 1 cup almond flour

3. 1 tsp sugar

4. 1 tsp salt

5. ½ tsp black pepper

6. 1 tsp baking powder

7. 5 sausages

8. 2 tsp olive oil

9. 1 tsp vanilla extract

10. ½ cup milk

Instructions:

- Preheat the oven at 325°F.

- Prepare a muffin tray having four compartments. Brush the muffin tray with olive oil.

- In a mixing bowl whisk the eggs and add milk. Mix well and add the vanilla extract.

- In a separate bowl mix all the dry ingredients.

- Now add the dry ingredients to the egg batter. Mix with a wooden spoon till a silky mixture is formed.

- Scoop out the batter from the bowl and pour in the muffin tray.

- Cut the sausages into small cubes.

- Top the batter in the muffin stray with sausages and bake for 20 minutes.

- When the muffins are baked, serve warm.

2.16. Almond Pancakes

Having pancakes on the weekends is always fun. But when you are following intermittent fasting you cannot consume a high amount of carbohydrates presents in the pancakes. In this pancake we have used almond flour.

- Total Time: 15 mins

- Prep Time: 10 mins

- Cooking Time: 5 mins

- Serving Size: 2-3 servings

Ingredients:

1. 2 eggs
2. 1 cup almond flour
3. 1 tsp honey
4. 1 tsp vanilla essence
5. 4/4 cup milk
6. Oil Spray

Instructions:

- In a mixing bowl, whisk the eggs and mix honey, vanilla essence, and milk.

- Fold the almond flour into the mixture and make a silky mixture.

- Spray the frying pan with oil and pour 1 large spoon of batter into the frying pan.

- Turn on the flame and cook for one minute on one side and then flip the pancake. Cook for one minute on the other side.

- Repeat the procedure with the entire batter.

- Serve with maple syrup or honey.

2.17. Veggie Omelet

This recipe is simple and delicious. You can make it every day or occasionally. Depends on your liking for eggs and fresh vegetables.

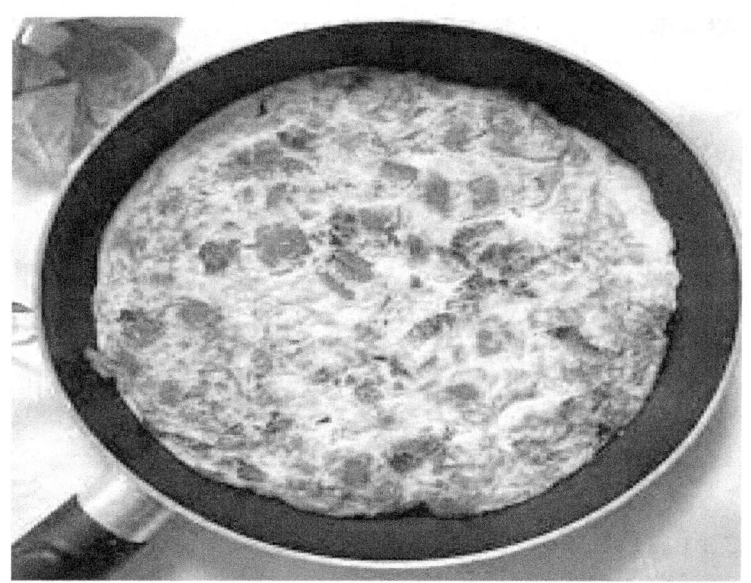

- Total Time: 15 mins

- Prep. Time: 10 mins

- Cooking Time: 5 mins

- Serving Size: 2 servings

Ingredients:

1. 3 eggs

2. ¼ tsp salt

3. ¼ tsp pepper

4. 1 small onion chopped.

5. 1 tomato chopped and seeds removed.

6. ½ green bell pepper chopped.

7. 1 green chili chopped.

8. ½ bunch coriander chopped.

9. 2 tbsp olive oil

Instructions:

- Whisk the eggs in the mixing bowl.

- Mix all the vegetables in the egg mixture.

- Add the salt and pepper.

- Mix well.

- In a frying pan add the olive oil and heat the pan at medium flame.

- Pour the batter into the pan and cook on each side for 3 minutes each.

- Take out on plate.

- Enjoy as it is or with a piece of toast.

2.18. Quiche

This is a delicious recipe for breakfast. It can be stored in a fridge for 3 to 4 days.

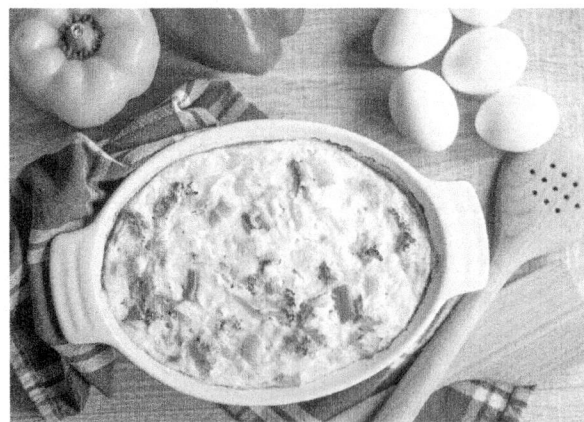

- Total Time: 1 hour

- Prep. Time: 10 mins

- Cooking Time: 45 mins

- Serving Size: 2-3 servings

Ingredients:

1. 4 eggs

2. 1 store bought pie crust.

3. 1 cup grated cheddar cheese.

4. 1 onion diced.

5. 1 bell pepper sliced.

6. 1 tomato diced.

7. ½ tsp salt

8. 1.2 tsp pepper

Instructions:

- Preheat the oven at 325∘F.

- Grease a casserole dish with olive oil.

- Set the pie crust at the bottom of the casserole dish.

- In a large mixing bowl, whisk eggs and add salt, pepper, and the vegetables and mix well.

- On the crust, put a layer of cheddar cheese.

- Then pour half of the egg batter.

- Next again, sprinkle a layer of cheese and then pour the remaining egg batter.

- Bake for 40 mins.

- Cut triangular pieces and serve warm.

2.19. French Toast

This is a sweet breakfast option that takes only a few minutes to make. It is a simple recipe with minimum ingredients.

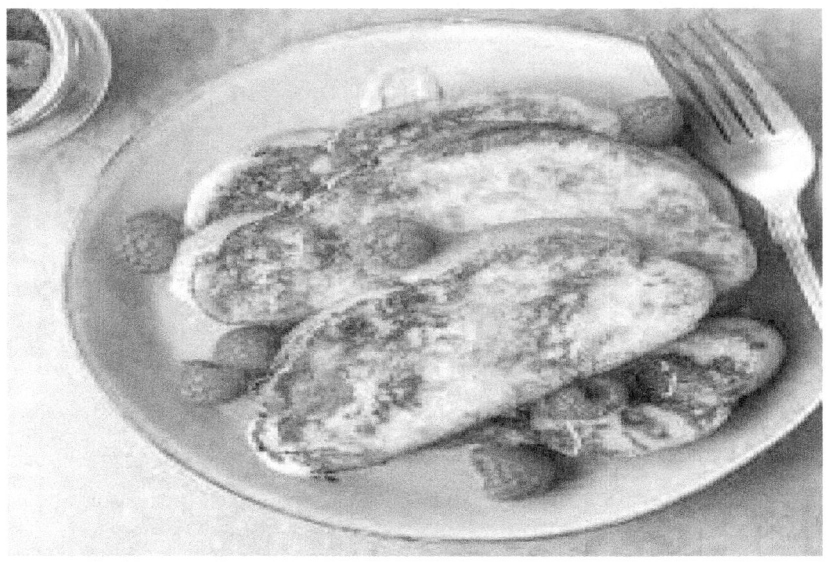

- Total Time: 15 mins

- Prep. Time: 10 mins

- Cooking Time: 5 mins

- Serving Size: 2 servings

Ingredients:

1. 2 eggs

2. 4 bread slices

3. ¼ cup milk

4. ¼ tsp cinnamon

5. 1 tsp sugar

6. 2 tbsp olive oil

Instructions:

- In a mixing bowl, mix all the ingredients except for the bread slices.

- Put olive oil in a frying pan and heat the frying pan with medium flame.

- Dip the bread slices in the egg batter on both sides and fry the bread slices.

- Cook the bread for 1 minute each on both sides.

- Serve with maple syrup or honey.

2.20. Chicken and Egg Wraps

This is a delicious recipe that is rich in protein. This is a simple recipe that can be made in under 20 minutes.

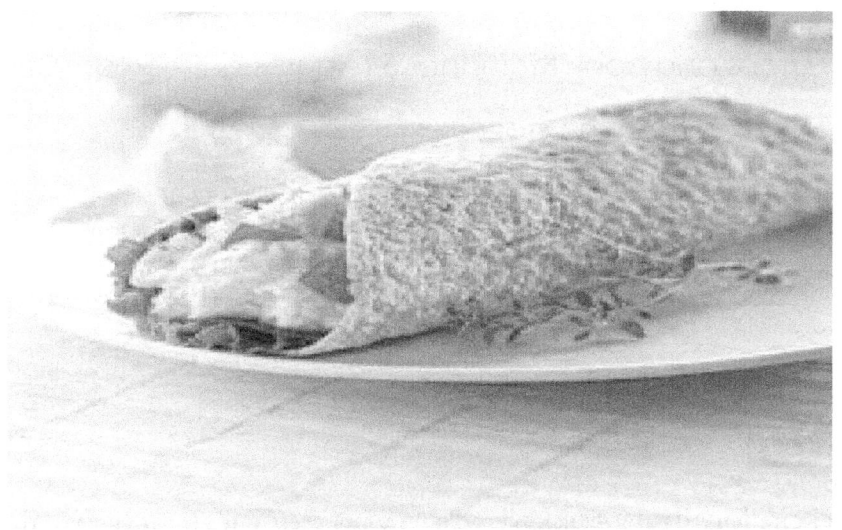

- Total Time: 30 mins

- Prep. Time: 15 mins

- Cooking Time: 15 mins

- Serving Size: 2 servings

Ingredients:

1. 3 large eggs

2. 1 chicken fillet cut into small cubes.

3. 1 tsp salt

4. 1 tsp pepper

5. 1 tsp minced garlic

6. 1 small onion chopped.

7. 1 small tomato chopped.

8. 2 whole-wheat wraps

9. ¼ cup olive oil

Instructions:

- In a frying pan, put 2 tbsp olive oil and crackle garlic in the pan.

- Add the onions and cook for 2 minutes. Then add the chicken, salt, and pepper.

- Cook for 4 to 5 mins.

- Add the tomatoes and cook for further 5 minutes on medium flame.

- Take off the chicken from the stove.

- Next, whisk the eggs and scramble them in a frying pan.

- Put both the fillings in the wraps and fold them.

- Serve warm.

2.21. Oatmeal

Oatmeal is a good option for breakfast when you decide to follow intermittent fasting. It gives you energy and strength, and kick-starts your day.

- Total Time: 10 mins

- Prep. Time: 5 mins

- Cooking Time: 5 mins

- Serving Size: 1 serving

Ingredients:

1. 2 tbsp quick oats

2. 1 cup milk

3. 1 tsp raisins

4. ½ tsp chia seeds

5. ½ tsp flax seeds

Instructions:

- In a saucepan put the milk and oats and bring them to a boil. Lower the flame and cook for 3 minutes.
- Take out the milk and oats in a cereal bowl.
- Top with the remaining ingredients.

2.22. Healthy Cereal Bowl

This is an easy and simple recipe for cereal. It has fresh fruit that will kick-start your day.

- Total Time: 10 mins
- Prep. Time: 5 mins
- Cooking Time: N/A
- Serving Size: 1 serving

Ingredients:

1. 1 cup milk
2. 5 tbsp cereal
3. 1 tsp honey
4. 2 strawberries sliced.
5. 3 blueberries
6. ½ tsp flax seeds
7. ½ tsp chia seeds

Instructions:

- In a cereal bowl, arrange the cereal, honey, strawberries, blueberries, chia seeds and flax seeds.
- Pour cold milk over the cereal.
- Enjoy your healthy cereal bowl.

2.23. Savory Oats

Some people do not have a sweet tooth and prefer savory oats. This recipe is just for those people.

- Total Time: 15 mins
- Prep. Time: 10 mins
- Cooking Time: 5 mins
- Serving Size: 1 serving

Ingredients:

1. 3 tbsp quick oats
2. 1 cup chicken broth
3. 100 g boiled chicken shredded.
4. ½ tsp salt
5. ½ tsp pepper
6. 2tsp lemon juice

Instructions:

- In a saucepan add the chicken broth and oats and cook for 5 mins.
- After that takeout in a cereal bowl and top with chicken, salt, pepper, and lemon juice.
- Enjoy the savory oatmeal.

2.24. Sunny Side up

This is the simplest recipe for a fried egg with brown bread.

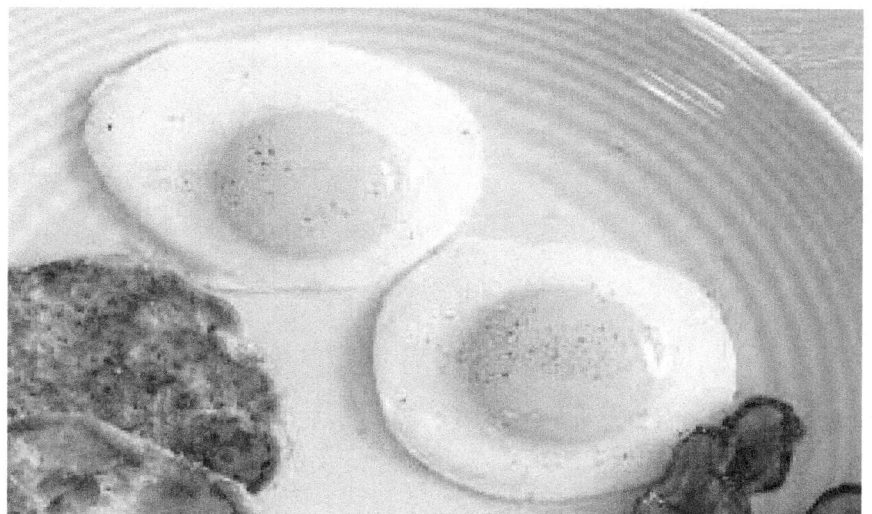

- Total Time: 5 mins

- Prep. Time: N/A

- Cooking time: 5 mins

- Serving Size: 1 serving

Ingredients:

1. 2 eggs

2. 1 pinch salt

3. 1 pinch pepper

4. 2 slices brown bread

5. 3 tbsp olive oil

Instructions:

- In a frying pan pours the olive oil and turn on the flame.

- Break both eggs in the pan and let them cook for 2 minutes.

- After 2 minutes, turn off the flame.

- Take the eggs out on a plate and garnish them with salt and pepper.

- Toast the bread slices and serve with eggs.

2.25. Creamy Mushrooms

Mushrooms are a great source of protein and cream is a good source of fat and dairy. This recipe is perfect to break your intermittent fast.

- Total Time: 10 mins
- Prep. Time: 5 mins
- Cooking time: 5 mins
- Serving Size: 2 servings

Ingredients:

1. 200g button mushrooms sliced.
2. 1 small onion sliced.
3. 1 small carrot diced.
4. ¼ tsp salt
5. ¼ tsp pepper
6. 1 tsp olive oil
7. ½ cup cream

Instructions:

- In a frying pan put the oil and onions and cook for 2 mins. Next, add the carrots and fry for 3 more minutes. Add water if required.
- Next, add the sliced mushrooms and cook for 3 mins.
- Take out the mushrooms and veggies on the plate.
- Garnish with salt and pepper.
- Top with fresh cream.

2.26. Fetta and Spinach Frittata

- Total Time: 45mins
- Prep. Time: 20 mins
- Cooking Time: 25 mins

- Serving Size: 8-10 servings

Ingredients:

1. 1 potato diced in 1/2-inch cubes.
2. 12 eggs
3. 2 tbsp olive oil
4. 200g spinach
5. 1 cup green onion chopped.
6. 1 cup feta cheese
7. 1 cup shredded cheddar or mozzarella cheese
8. ¾ cup cream
9. ½ teaspoon black pepper
10. Salt to taste
11. Olive oil

Instructions:

- Preheat the oven to 400 °F.
- Sauté the spinach until it is wilted in a wide pan, rinse and strain out the juice.
- Add potatoes with little olive oil until soft and slightly brown. Add black pepper and salt and cook for 10 to 15 minutes. Let the vegetables cool.
- To a separate bowl, beat eggs, milk, pepper, and salt until a smooth mixture is formed. Add cheese and onions. Combine and fold in the potato and spinach.
- Heat oil in a bake-proof pan. Add the frittata mixture to the pan and cook it till it starts to set.
- Put it in the oven and bake for 15 to 20 minutes.
- Serve while warm.

2.27. Sausage and Potato Frittata

- Total Time: 40 mins
- Prep. Time: 20 mins
- Cooking Time: 20 mins
- Serving Size: 8 servings

Ingredients:

1. 4 sausages (any meat) cut into ½ inch pieces.
2. 12 large eggs, lightly beaten.
3. 1 Yukon potato cut into ¼" slices.
4. 1 tbsp olive oil
5. 1/2 cup cream
6. 1 cup shredded mozzarella
7. 1 cup grated parmesan cheese.
8. 5 tsp thinly sliced green onion.
9. 1 tsp salt
10. 1 tsp pepper
11. Salsa or sour cream (optional)

Instructions:

- Preheat to 400 °F.
- Use a sauté pan to cook bits of sausage until cooked. Take out and place on a kitchen towel to lose any moisture left.
- Now cook the potato with olive oil until soft and slightly brown. Leave it to cool. Beat the eggs. Add milk, salt, and pepper in a bowl until a fluffy mixture is formed.
- Add in the cheese and onion. Fold in the potatoes and sausages.
- Heat olive oil on a stove in a 10-inch ovenproof pan. Mix the frittata batter thoroughly and add to the pan. Cook it till the frittata is set at the bottom.

- Place the pan in the oven. Bake for 15-20 mins.

- Serve while hot.

2.28. Healthy Omelet

- Total time: 20 mins

- Prep. Time: 5 mins

- Cooking Time: 15mins

- Serving size: 3 servings

Ingredients:

1. 8 large eggs

2. 1 tsp salt

3. 3 tbsp sour cream

4. 1.5 tsp butter

5. ½ cup milk

6. 2 chopped green onions.

Instructions:

- Preheat the oven at 325 °F. Use butter to grease a medium baking pan.

- In a large bowl, beat the eggs, salt, and milk until mixed.

- Stir together the green onions.

- Pour this mixture into the baking pan already prepared.

- Bake the batter until set. It takes 25-30 minutes to fully cook.

- Sprinkle the remaining cheese over the eggs, continue to bake for another 3-4 minutes, and wait for the cheese to melt.

2.29. Fluffy Pan Cakes

- Total time: 20 mins

- Prep time: 10 mins

- Cooking time: 10 mins

- Serving Size: 4 servings

Ingredients:

1. 4 large eggs

2. ¾ cup flour

3. 4 tablespoon butter (melted)

4. ¾ cup milk

5. ¼ tsp salt

6. 1 ½ tbsp sugar

Instructions:

- Before anything else, preheat the oven to 375 °F.

- Grease a baking pan. Use a medium-size flat pan.

- To make a smooth batter, beat all the eggs in a mixing bowl, then put in butter, milk, sugar, and salt.

- Whisk for 5 minutes to get a fluffy batter.

- Add the flour in sections and fold into the batter. This way, no lumps are formed.

- Slowly pour into the baking pan and put to bake.

- Bake it for 8-12 minutes.

- Test for doneness. Take out when the batter is set.

- Serve warm with maple syrup and a choice of fresh fruits.

2.30. French toast in an Oven

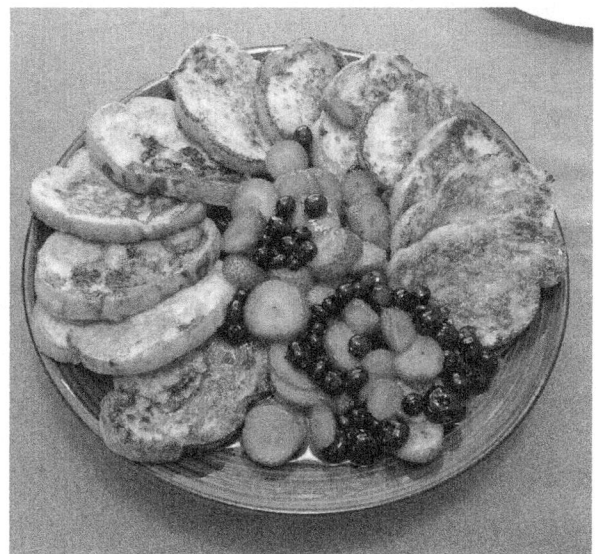

- Total Time: 1 hour 30 mins

- Prep time: 40mins

- Cooking time: 10mins

- Serving size: 2 servings

Ingredients:

1. 2/3 a cup of milk

2. 1 tsp of ground cinnamon

3. 1/2 cup of sugar

4. 4 eggs

5. 1/2 tsp of table salt

6. 2 tsp vanilla essence (or a scraped vanilla bean)

7. 1 white bread loaf

8. ½ cup of milk

Instructions:

- Cut white bread loaf into thick slices. The slices should be thick enough to soak in the custard.

- Mix the milk, sugar, cream, salt, vanilla essence, and ground cinnamon.

- Whisk well to form a smooth custard-like batter.

- Arrange a rimmed dish with bread slices. On the slices, pour custard.

- Let the custard soak for 25 minutes, then flip the slices after 10 minutes to ensure soaking evenly. Be sure that the custard soaks to the center as well as the corners of the slices.

- You might even let the entire tray soak in the refrigerator overnight.

- Now, line a baking dish with butter paper. Shift the soaked slices to the prepared baking dish, arranging that there is a little gap between the slices.

- Bake for 25 to 30minutes at 300 °F.

- After 30 minutes, check the dish. The slices should be soft but be sure that they are not soggy. If they are still wet, bake for another 5 minutes.

- Serve with fresh fruits.

- Serve hot.

2.31. French toast in a Casserole

- Total Time: 1 hour

- Prep. Time: 15 minutes

- Cooking Time: 45 minutes

- Serving size: 3 servings

Ingredients:

1. 2 1/2 cup milk

2. 2 tbsp pure maple syrup or brown sugar.

3. 1/2 tsp Cinnamon powder

4. 2 tsp of vanilla essence

5. salt to taste

6. 6 Eggs

7. 1 loaf of bread

8. 3 tbsp unsalted butter

9. 2 tbsp of brown sugar or maple syrup.

Instructions:

- Preheat the oven at 350 °F.

- Spray an 11-inch by 11-inch dish evenly with cooking oil or butter.

- Cut the bread slices into small 2-inch by 2-inch cubes. Place these in an even layer.

- Whisk the eggs, one tablespoon of pure maple syrup, cinnamon powder, vanilla essence, and salt in a large bowl.

- Now, spread the mixture generously over the bread.

- Stir the melted butter, cinnamon powder, and maple syrup in a smaller bowl. Drizzle this dressing on the casserole.

- (You could refrigerate this casserole overnight with a cling wrap at this stage and bake in the morning or put it in the fridge for 15-20 minutes and bake).

- Use a foil sheet to cover the dish and bake it for 30 minutes.

- Remove the foil and cook for another 15-20 minutes, until the bread is slightly browned at the top.

- Serve with fruit of choice and maple syrup.

2.32. Coco Pancakes

- Total Time: 20 mins

- Prep. Time: 10 mins

- Cooking Time: 10 mins

- Serving Size: 2 servings

Ingredients:

1. 1 ripe banana

2. ½ cup almond flour

3. 1 tsp coco powder

4. 1 egg

5. ¼ cup milk

6. 2 tbsp olive oil

Instructions:

- Mash the ripe banana and mix all the ingredients to make a smooth batter.

- If the batter is thick add a bit more milk.

- Heat olive oil in a pan.

- Pour 2 tbsp of batter in the pan and spread into a circular shape.

- Cook on one side for 1 minute and flip. Cook on another side for 30 seconds.

- Take off from the heat and put on a serving plate.

- Repeat the whole procedure with the entire batter.

- Serve with maple sauce.

Chapter 3.

Snacks and Salads

When you follow intermittent fasting, it is recommended to include snacks and salads in your diet. Another important consideration is that healthy and energy-packed snacks should be consumed rather than junk food when you start following a healthy routine. Another aim of intermittent fasting is to keep insulin levels in check. In this chapter, you will find all snacks and salads which ensure a minimum insulin spike.

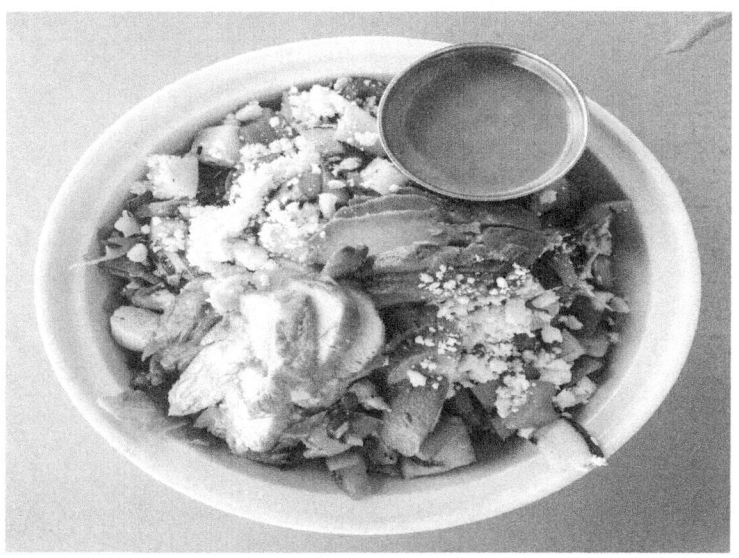

3.1. Healthy Trail Mix

This is a perfect snack when you are at work or on the go. It is simple to prepare and can easily be stored for 1 to 2 months if kept properly in an airtight container. You can also make small packets to keep in your work bag or purse. They give you an instant energy boost when you experience an energy dip during the day.

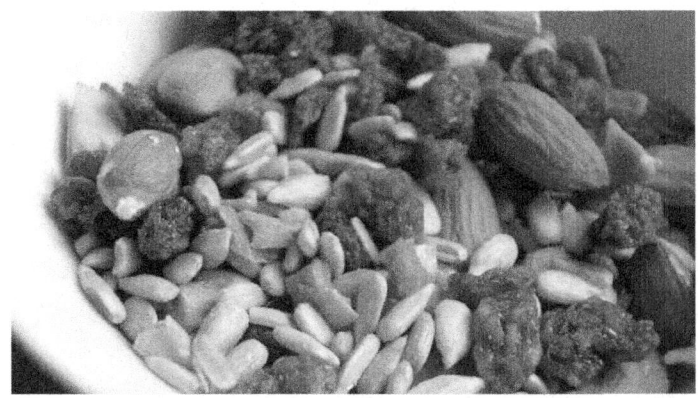

- Total Time: 5-10 mins

- Prep. Time: 5-10 mins

- Cook Time: N/A

- Serving Size: 10-12 servings

Ingredients:

1. ¼ cup coconut shavings

2. 1 cup almonds

3. ½ cup raisins

4. 1 cup raw sunflower seeds

5. ½ cup dried apricots (chopped)

6. ¼ cup chocolate chips

Instructions:

- In a large container, put in all the ingredients.

- Mix them well and transfer them to an airtight container.

- It can be kept for 1 to 2 months.

- It can be stored by keeping a fist full in zip lock bags and storing them.

3.2. Prawn Salad

Another healthy option for women to consume protein is seafood. This is a simple prawn salad recipe that you can take as a snack. The recipe has avocado as well, which serves as an excellent fat source. Avocadoes provide good fat and are extremely beneficial for brain health.

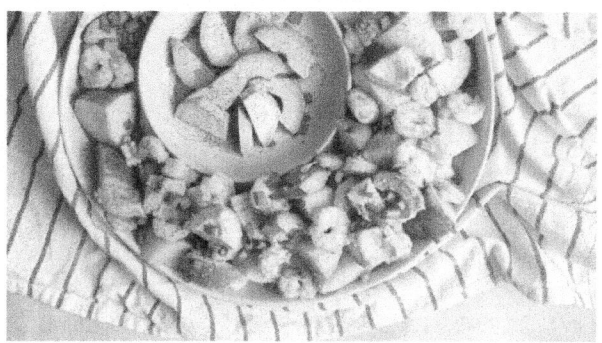

- Total Time: 30 mins

- Prep. Time: 10 mins

- Cook Time: 20 Mins

- Serving Size: 2 servings

Ingredients:

1. 1 ripe avocado

2. 300 g potatoes

3. 250 grams jumbo prawns

4. 2 spring onions chopped.

5. 1 tbsp Cajun seasoning

6. 2 tsp olive oil

7. 1 clove garlic minced.

8. 1 tsp salt

9. 1 cup alfalfa sprouts

Instructions:

- In a large saucepan, pour water and put in the potatoes. Put in 1 tsp salt and boil the potatoes till cooked.

- When the potatoes are cooked, let them cool. Then peel and dice into cubes.

- If you have deveined and peeled prawns, this step can be skipped. Otherwise, peel and devein the prawns. Bring water to boil in a medium-sized pan and put in the prawns. Let them stay for 5 minutes and take them out. Towel-dry the prawns.

- In a frying pan, add the garlic, prawns, spring onion, and Cajun seasoning and cook over medium flame for 2 minutes. Add the potatoes and toss for 1 to 2 mins.

- Take the salad out on a salad bowl.

- Peal and dice an avocado. Top the salad with avocado and alfalfa sprouts.

- Serve cold.

3.3. Mediterranean Salad

This recipe is a Mediterranean salad with quinoa. Quinoa is a super food and helps keep insulin levels low and provides protein for the body.

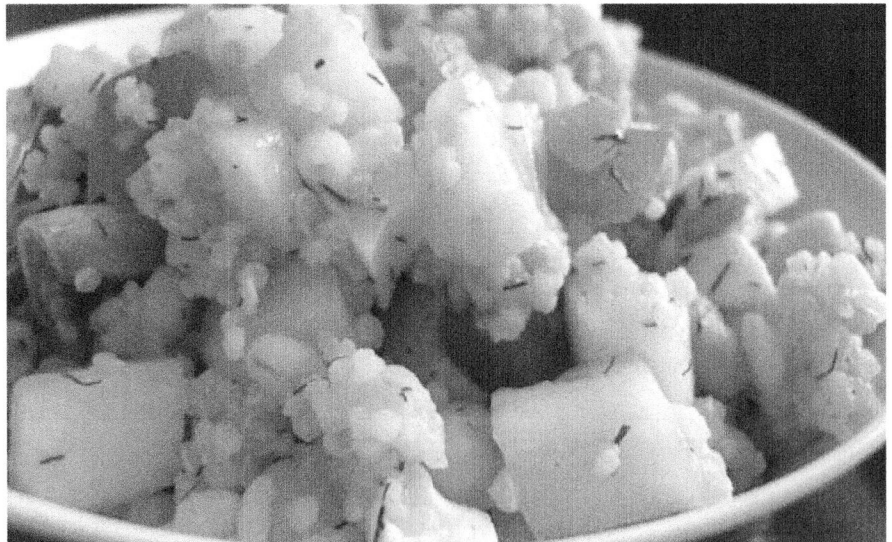

- Total Time: 25 mins

- Prep. Time: 10 mins

- Cook Time: 15 mins

- Serving Size: 2 -3 servings

Ingredients:

1. ½ cup white quinoa
2. 1 cup millet
3. 2 cup water
4. 1 tomato diced and seeds removed.
5. 1 cucumber diced.
6. 1 red onion thinly chopped,
7. 200g feta cheese
8. 200 g white beans can drain.
9. ½ tsp cayenne pepper
10. ½ tsp ground pepper
11. 1 red bell pepper seeded and diced.
12. ¼ cup pine nuts peeled.

Instructions:

- In a saucepan, put in quinoa with ¾ cup of water. Bring to boil, and then lower the flame. Let it simmer for 5 mins and take off from the flame. Let it stay for 10 mins.

- In another saucepan, put in millet and 1 cup water. Bring to boil and lower flame. Let it simmer for 10 mins. Keep aside for 10 mins.

- In a large salad bowl, put in the millet and quinoa. Mix in all the remaining ingredients and toss.

- The salad is ready to eat.

3.4. Chickpeas Salad

This is a tangy-flavored chickpea salad. You can eat this for your snack time during your eating window.

- Total Time: 20 mins

- Prep. Time: 20 mins
- Cooking Time: N/A
- Serving Size: 2 servings

Ingredients:

1. 200 g cooked chickpeas
2. 1 small onion chopped.
3. 1 potato boiled and cubed.
4. 1 tomato chopped.
5. ½ tsp salt
6. ½ tsp red chili powder
7. 2 tsp tamarind pulp

Instructions:

- Cut and prepare all the ingredients.
- In a large mixing bowl, add all the ingredients and mix well.
- Your chickpea salad is ready to serve.

3.5. Kidney Bean Salad

This salad is a simple salad with few ingredients and can easily be made in under 15 minutes. It is a perfect option for snack time.

- Total Time: 15 mins
- Prep. Time: 15 mins
- Cooking Time: N/A
- Serving Size: 2 servings

Ingredients:

1. 200g cooked kidney beans
2. 1 small onion chopped.

3. 1 tomato chopped.

4. 100g cilantro chopped.

5. 2 tbsp tomato ketchup

Instructions:

- Cut and prepare all the ingredients.

- In a large mixing bowl, add all the ingredients and mix well.

- Your chickpea salad is ready to serve.

3.6. Grilled Chicken Salad

When you follow intermittent fasting, one important thing is that you reduce your carbohydrate intake so that your fat-burning system is triggered. But if you reduce carbohydrates, you will feel hungry at shorter intervals. To fill the void, it is recommended to eat a large protein portion with all your meals. This chicken salad will give you a good protein portion.

- Total Time: 30 mins

- Prep Time: 10 mins

- Cooking Time: 15 mins

- Serving Size: 2 servings

Ingredients:

1. 2 skinless chicken breasts

2. 2 tbsp Olive oil

3. 1 tsp salt

4. 2 tbsp vinegar

5. 1/2 tsp pepper

6. 1 bunch salad leaves

7. 1 onion sliced.

8. 1 tomato sliced.

9. 2 tbsp Italian salad dressing

Instructions:

- In a small bowl, mix vinegar, salt, and pepper.
- Rub this mixture on the chicken breast pieces.
- Warm a stove grill and brush it lightly with olive oil.
- Put the chicken breasts on the grill.
- Cook on a medium flame for 7 minutes on each side. And additional two minutes on each side.
- Take off the chicken from the flame and cut diagonally.
- In a mixing bowl, add all the fresh vegetables.
- IN the bowl, add the chicken and top with Italian dressing and the remaining olive oil.
- Serve at room temperature.

3.7. Farro Salad

Another special recipe for your snack time. The instructions are easy to follow, and be sure that you are in for a delicious salad.

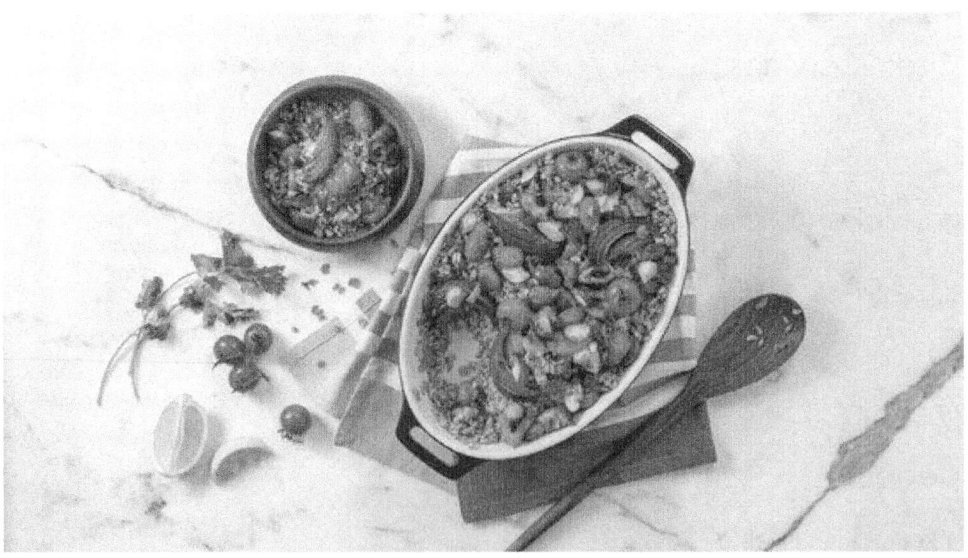

- Total Time: 1 hour
- Prep. Time: 15 mins

- Cooking Time: 45 mins
- Serving Size: 4 servings

Ingredients:

1. 1 cup farro
2. 2 cup almond milk
3. 1 eggplant diced.
4. 1 zucchini diced.
5. 1 medium onion cut in wedges.
6. 6 garlic cloves sliced.
7. 3 tbsp olive oil
8. 1 tsp salt
9. ½ tsp pepper
10. Balsamic vinegar
11. Green onion chopped for garnish.

Instructions:

- Preheat oven at 325°F.
- On butter, paper, spread the eggplant and rub salt on it. The eggplant will leave the water. Squeeze the eggplant in a paper towel to remove excess water.
- IN a large mixing bowl, mix the onion, zucchini, and eggplant. Drizzle 1 tbsp olive oil and toss the vegetables.
- Prepare a baking tray with butter paper and spread the vegetables.
- Bake for 20 minutes.
- Meanwhile, wash and drain the farro. IN a large saucepan, pour almond milk and add farro. Bring to boil, and then lower the flame. Let the farro simmer for 15 minutes, and then off the flame. Let the farro remain in the saucepan for five minutes.
- Next, dish out the farro on a plate and top it with the vegetables. Olive oil, balsamic salt, and spring onions.
- Serve at room temperature.

3.8. Black Bean Soup

This is an energy-packed soup with proteins and dietary fiber. This soup is perfect for a winter evening.

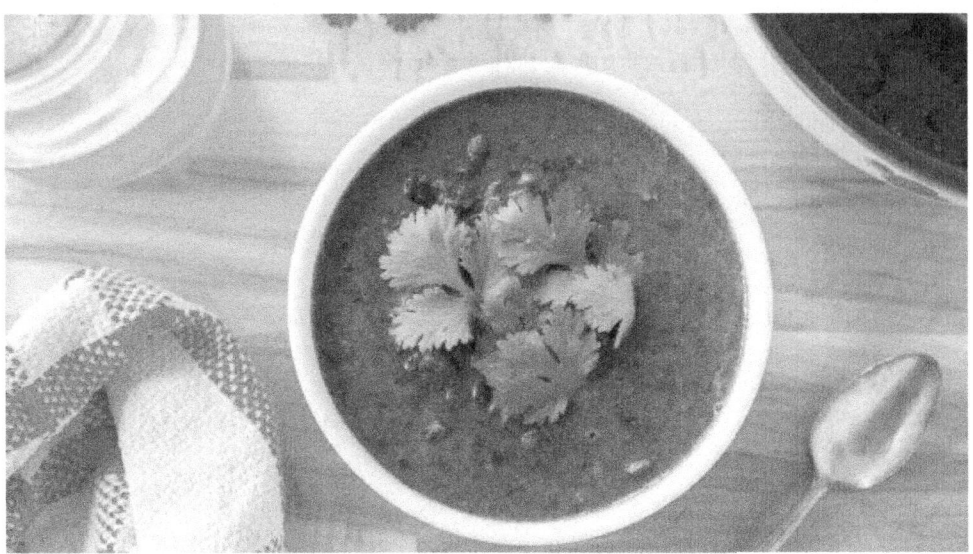

- Total Time: 30 mins
- Prep. Time: 5 mins
- Cooking Time: 25 mins
- Serving Size: 4 servings

Ingredients:

1. 600 g black beans cooked.
2. 3 tbsp olive oil
3. 1 onion chopped.
4. 1 tsp cumin powder
5. 2 sliced garlic cloves
6. ½ tsp salt
7. ½ tsp red pepper
8. 2 cups chicken or vegetable broth
9. Cilantro for garnish

Instructions:

- In a medium-size pot, add the oil and onion. Fry the onion till it becomes translucent.
- Add cumin powder and cook for 1 minute.
- Next, add garlic and cook for 30 seconds more.
- Next, add half of the black beans and chicken broth with salt and pepper.
- Cook for 20 mins.
- Next, put the whole mixture in a blender and blend to form a smooth soup.
- Please put it back in the pot and add the remaining beans. Cook for 5 more minutes and pour into serving bowls.
- Garnish with cilantro.
- Serve hot.

3.9. Potato Crisps

Potato crisps are a guilty pleasure for most of us. But due to the high content of oil and carbohydrate, most of us avoid it. But during intermittent fasting, no foods are off-limits. These crisps are good to curb your craving for chips.

- Total Time: 20 mins
- Prep. Time: 5 mins
- Cooking Time: 15 mins
- Serving Size: 1 serving

Ingredients:

1. 1 tsp olive oil
2. 1 large potato
3. 1 pinch salt
4. 1 pinch pepper

Instructions:

- Wash the potato and slice it thinly.

- Preheat oven at 325°F.

- Prepare a baking sheet with butter paper.

- Spread the potato slices on the sheet.

- Brush the slices with olive oil and sprinkle salt and pepper.

- Bake for 15 minutes.

- Serve warm and can also be stored for 2 weeks.

3.10. Baked Potato

This is a wonderful recipe. This recipe uses olive oil, which gives extra flavor. You can eat it as a snack or can be used as a dinner option for intermittent fasting.

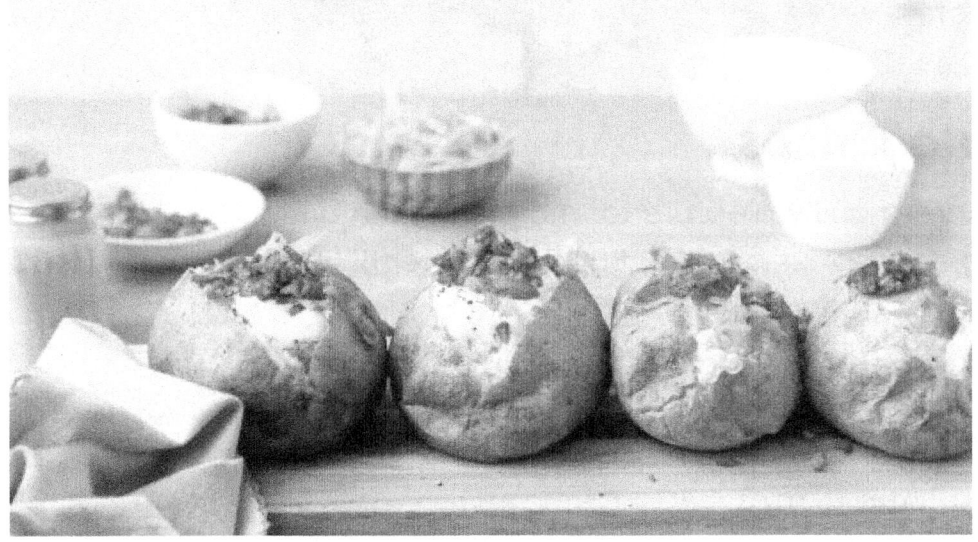

- Total Time: 1 hour

- Prep Time: 5 mins

- Cooking Time: 55 min

- Serving Size: 1 person

Ingredients:

1. 1 large potato

2. ½ tsp kosher salt

3. 2 tbsp olive oil

Instructions:

- Wash the potato and then dry it. Poke it deeply with a fork at 8 to 12 places.

- Preheat oven to 300◦F.

- Prepare a baking tray with butter paper.

- Rub the potato with oil and then salt.

- Bake for 55 mins. Take out. The skin should be crisp, but the potato inside should be soft.

- You can eat it as it is by removing the skin or can make a cut in the potato and fill it with toppings of your choice.

3.11. Cauliflower Snack

This snack is a great alternative to regular popcorn. You can even call it cauliflower popcorn.

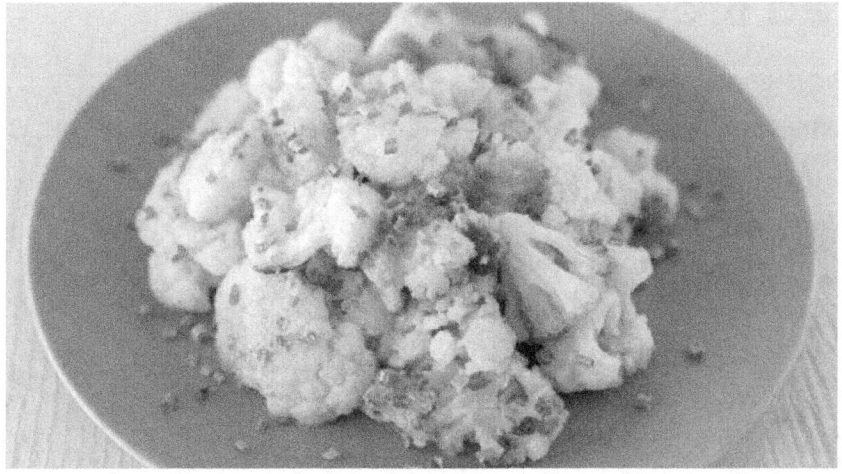

- Total Time: 1 hour

- Prep Time: 5 mins

- Cooking Time: 55 mins

- Serving Size: 1-2 servings

Ingredients:

1. 1 cauliflower head

2. ½ tsp salt

3. 2 tbsp olive oil

Instructions:

- Preheat oven to 400◦F.

- Prepare a baking sheet with butter paper.

- Cut the florets of the cauliflower into small pieces. Remove the thick stems and the core.

- In a mixing bowl, whisk the olive oil and salt.

- Add the florets and toss them well.

- Spread the cauliflower on the tray.

- Bake for 55 mins.

- Eat immediately because this cannot be kept for a long while.

3.12. Roasted Broccoli

This is a good option for snacking because it is packed with energy and flavor. It keeps your insulin levels stable and does not give an unnecessary spike which you experience with most store-bought snacks.

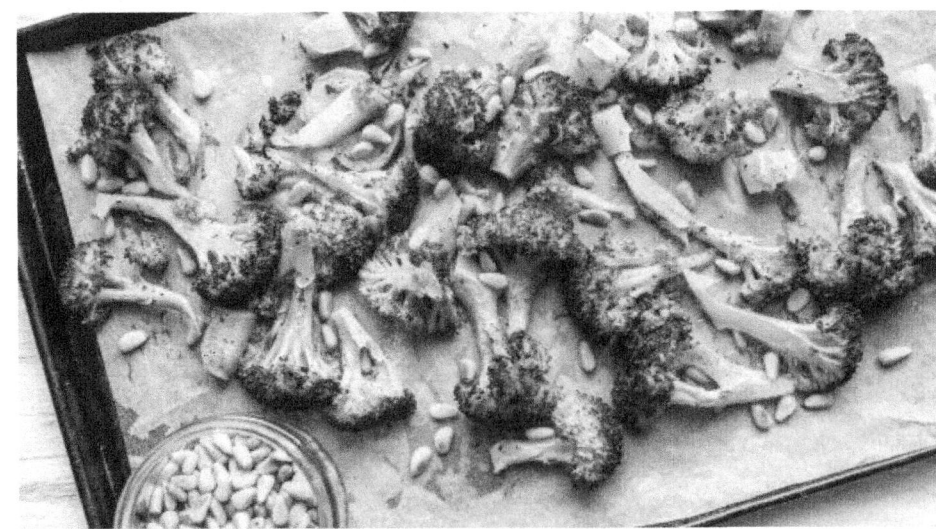

- Total Time: 20 mins

- Prep. Time: 8 mins

- Cooking Time: 12 mins

- Serving Size: 2 servings

Ingredients:

1. 500g broccoli florets
2. 2 tbsp olive oil
3. 2 tbsp pine nuts
4. ¼ tsp salt
5. ¼ tsp pepper
6. 2 tbsp butter
7. 1 tsp lemon zest
8. 2 tbsp lemon juice

Instructions:

- Preheat the oven to 500∘F.
- Prepare a baking sheet with butter paper.
- In a large bowl, out the broccoli florets and toss them with olive oil, salt, and pepper.
- Spread them on a baking tray and bake for 12 minutes.
- Please put them in a salad bowl.
- In a saucepan, melt the butter and add lemon zest and lemon juice to the butter.
- Drizzle the butter on the broccoli and top with pine nuts.

3.13. Apple and Potato Salad

This salad is simple to prepare and is a wonderful snack to eat.

- Total Time: 20 mins
- Prep. Time: 5 mins
- Cooking Time: 10 mins
- Serving Size: 1 serving

Ingredients:

1. 1 apple
2. 1 potato
3. 1 tsp lemon juice
4. 1 tsp mustard
5. ¼ tsp salt
6. ¼ tsp pepper
7. 1 tbsp olive oil
8. ¼ tsp rosemary

Instructions:

- Remove the apple seeds and dice them, and put them in a mixing bowl.
- Boil the potato. Peel it and dice it into cubes. Mix with the apples.
- A small bowl makes a dressing by mixing the remaining ingredients and drizzle over the apples and potato.
- Enjoy your cold salad.

3.14. Coleslaw

This is a simple recipe with few ingredients and a lovely flavor. This is one of the most simple and delicious salads.

- Total Time: 10 mins
- Prep. Time: 5 mins
- Cooking Time: N/A
- Serving Size: 2 servings

Ingredients:

1. 100 g green cabbage chopped.
2. 100 g purple cabbage chopped.
3. 1 small carrot chopped.

4. 1 small onion chopped.

5. 2 tbsp cream

6. 2 tbsp mayonnaise

7. 1 pinch salt

8. 1 pinch pepper

Instructions:

- In a large mixing bowl, add all ingredients.

- Mix and toss the ingredients together.

- Enjoy your delicious salad.

3.15. Prawn Salad

Seafood salads are healthy and delicious. This salad recipe is easy to follow, and you will not regret it once you try this out.

- Total Time: 30 mins

- Prep. Time: 15 mins

- Cooking Time: 10 mins

- Serving Size: 1 serving

Ingredients:

1. 150 g prawns

2. 2 cup water

3. 1 tsp salt

4. 1 onion thinly sliced.

5. ½ bell pepper thinly sliced.

6. 1 tomato sliced.

7. ½ tsp pepper

8. 1 tbsp lemon juice

9. 1 tsp olive oil

Instructions:

- Remove the skins of the prawns and devein them. Wash with cold water.

- In 2 cups of water in a saucepan and bring to boil.

- Add the prawns to this water and let them boil for 5 mins.

- Please take out the prawns and dry them.

- In a large bowl, mix all ingredients and then drizzle olive oil and lemon juice.

3.16. Oven-Baked Potato Wedges

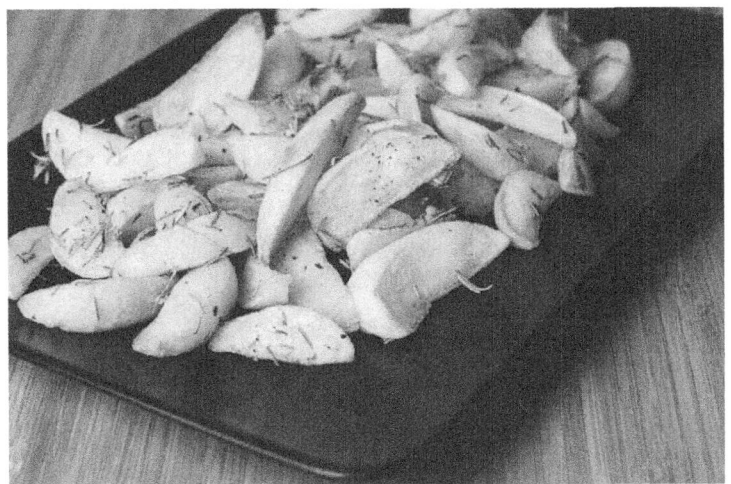

- Total Time: 40 mins

- Prep. time: 5 mins

- Cook time: 35 mins.

- Serving size: 2-4 servings

Ingredients:

1. 200g potatoes

2. 2 tbsp olive oil

3. ½ tsp dried rosemary

4. Salt to taste

Instructions:

- First, preheat the oven to 350 °F.

- Prepare a baking tray by lining it with butter paper.

- Clean the potatoes thoroughly. Keep the skins.

- Cut the potatoes into wedges.

- In a large bowl, toss the potatoes with olive oil.

- Set the potatoes in the baking tray.

- Top the potatoes with rosemary and salt.

- Bake for 30-35 minutes or until the potato edges tend to brown.

- Take it out of the oven.

3.17. Baked Veggie Salad

- Total Time: 50 mins

- Prep Time: 10 mins

- Cook Time:40 mins

- Serving size: 6 servings

Ingredients:

1. 2 medium eggplants

2. 2 butternut squash

3. 2 large red peppers

4. 1 medium zucchini

5. 1 red onion

6. 100g feta cheese crumbled.

7. ½ cup olive oil

8. salt to taste

9. ½ teaspoon sugar

10. 1 teaspoon black pepper

11. 2 teaspoon mustard

12. 3 tablespoon balsamic vinegar

13. 2 ½ tablespoon fresh mint leaves chopped.

14. 1 ½ tablespoon chopped basil.

15. 2 garlic cloves chopped.

Instructions

- First, preheat the convection oven at 400 °F.

- Line two wide baking trays with butter paper.

- Place the vegetables in a mixing bowl, coat in oil, and season with pepper and salt.

- Arrange them on the baking trays in a single layer.

- Bake in the oven for 30 -40 minutes or a bit longer if you want a crispy finish.

- For the dressing, combine into a small container all the dressing components. Mix and season with pepper and salt.

- Place the vegetables on a platter for serving.

- Drizzle the dressing over it and check the Seasoning.

- Top it with feta cheese, basil, and mint leaves.

3.18. Yummy Seafood Bits

- Total Time: 5o mins

- Prep time: 10 mins

- Cook time: 40 mins.

- Serving size: 6 servings

Ingredients

1. 1 cup shrimp

2. 1 cup crab meat

3. 1 onion chopped.

4. 1 green bell pepper chopped.

5. 1 lemon

6. ¾ cup <u>mayonnaise</u>

7. 3 tbsp. butter

8. 2 tbsp <u>Worcestershire sauce</u>

9. <u>salt</u> to taste

10. ½ tsp <u>pepper</u>

11. ½ cup soft breadcrumbs

12. ½ tsp <u>paprika</u>

Instruction

- First, preheat the oven to 350 F.

- Use hands to flake the crab meat.

- Next, the crab meat, shrimp, mayonnaise, green pepper, celery, and cabbage are mixed in a bowl.

- In a small cup, combine pepper, salt, and Worcestershire sauce.

- Line a mini muffin tray.

- Scoop out the crab mixture and put it into the muffin compartments.

- Top with breadcrumbs. Drizzle with Worcestershire dressing.

- Bake for 30 minutes.

- After taking it out, top it with paprika and pepper to serve.

3.19. Baked Croutons

- Total Time: 15-20 mins

- Prep time: 5 mins

- Cooking time: 10-15 mins

- Serving size: 1 serving

Ingredients:

1. 2 slice French bread
2. 2 tsp parmesan cheese
3. 2 tsp olive oil
4. ½ tsp Italian Seasoning
5. Salt to taste

Instructions:

- First, preheat the oven to 325 ° F.
- Put the cooking rack of the oven at the bottom. Cut the bread slices into 1/2-inch squares.
- In a large bowl, add bread pieces and oil, then toss them. Add parmesan cheese, Italian dressing, and salt. Mix them so that bread pieces are nicely coated.
- Line a baking sheet with aluminum foil and spread cubes of bread on the baking sheet.
- Bake for 8 minutes. Turn the croutons over and bake for eight more minutes. Check if the croutons are light brown and crunchy. If not, bake for 2-3 minutes more.
- Pull out the baking sheet from the oven. Garnish with parmesan cheese and Italian dressing.
- Let the croutons cool before use.
- The croutons can be used immediately or can be kept for a week.

3.20. Cheese Crisps

- Total Time: 15 mins
- Prep time: 5 mins
- Cooking time: 10 mins
- Serving Size: 2 servings

Ingredients:

1. 7 tbsp shredded parmesan cheese

2. ½ tsp dried oregano

3. Salt to season

Instructions:

- Preheat the oven to 325 °F.

- Put the baking rack in the bottom position.

- Cover a baking tray with aluminum foil.

- Spoon the cheese on the tray in tablespoon-sized balls, keeping them 1 1/2 inches apart.

- Pat each cheese ball softly into the baking tray.

- Bake this for 5 minutes or until the cheese has melted and bubbles are formed.

- Take out the tray and sprinkle Seasoning.

- Put back the tray to the oven and bake for around 2-4 minutes until the center is no longer bubbly. The crisps should be soft and golden.

- Take out from the oven and let them cool before use.

- These can be stored for a week in an airtight container.

3.21. Sweet Potato Crisps

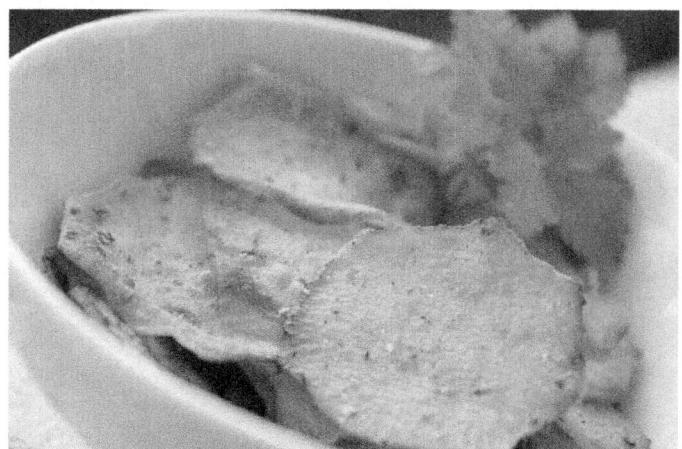

- Total Time: 20 mins

- Prep time: 10 mins

- Cooking time: 20 mins

Ingredients:

1. 200g sweet potatoes.

2. ½ tsp ground cinnamon

3. Salt to taste

4. 2 tbsp vegetable oil

Instructions:

- At the convection setting, preheat the oven at 400 ° F.

- Place the oven rack at the lowest position.

- Cover a baking tray with aluminum foil.

- Slice sweet potatoes too thin chips.

- Mix them with oil, cinnamon, and salt in a mixing bowl.

- Arrange sweet potato chips on the prepared pan in a single layer.

- For 10 minutes, bake sweet potato slices.

- Take them out of the oven, turn the slices over and bake for another 8 minutes.

- Take out of the oven when the sweet potatoes are slightly brown.

- Let them cool before serving.

3.22. Seafood Stuffed Peppers

- Total Time: 35 mins

- Prep time: 20 mins

- Cooking time: 15 mins

- Serving Size: 2 servings

Ingredients:

1. 2 green bell peppers

2. 12 prawns deveined and chopped.

3. 1 onion

4. 1 Medium Tomato

5. 1 tbsp chopped coriander leaves

6. 3 tbsp cream

7. 4 tbsp grated cheese

8. 2 tsp lemon juice

9. 3 tbsp olive oil

10. ½ tsp turmeric powder

11. 1 tsp red chili

12. ¼ tsp sugar

13. Salt to taste

Instructions:

- Preheat the oven to 325 °F.

- Prepare a baking sheet by lining it with butter paper.

- Cut the bell peppers in half and get rid of the seeds. Clean out the white membranes as well so that a pepper cup is formed.

- Rub a pinch of salt in each pepper cup.

- De-vein and wash the prawns. Get rid of the tails. Chop into tiny pieces.

- Add oil to a frying pan. Stir fry the onions and tomatoes until soft.

- Add the prawns and all other ingredients except for cream and coriander.

- Let it fry for 3 to 4 minutes, add the cream, and cook on low flame for two minutes.

- Take off the flame and add coriander.

- Fill the bell pepper cups with this filling.

- Arrange the bell pepper on the prepared baking sheet.

- Top them with cheese.

- Bake for 10 minutes or till the cheese is melted.

- Serve warm.

3.23. Chicken stuffed Mushrooms

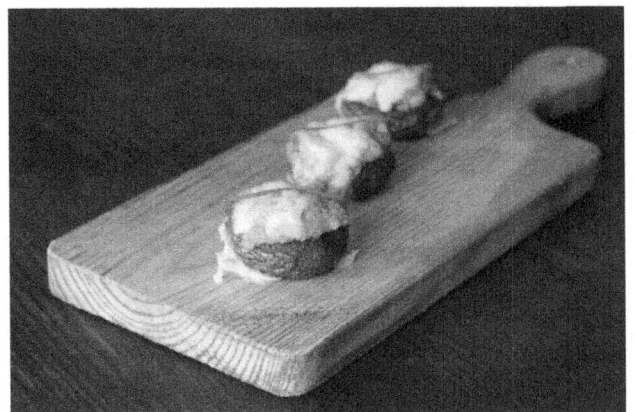

- Total Time: 45mins

- Prep time: 20 mins

- Cooking time: 25 mins

- Serving Size: 4 servings

Ingredients:

1. 20 mushrooms

2. 150g chicken mince

3. 2 green onions

4. 200g cream cheese

5. 2 tbsp mayonnaise

6. 4 tbsp cheddar cheese

7. 2 tbsp Parmesan cheese

8. 2 tbsp butter

9. 2 tsp hot sauce

10. 1/2 cup breadcrumbs

11. Salt to taste

12. ½ tsp pepper

Instructions:

- Preheat the oven to 400 ° F.

- Prepare a large baking tray by covering it with aluminum foil.

- Combine the cream cheese, mayonnaise, and both types of cheese with an electric mixer.

- Fold the salt, hot sauce, vinegar, onions, and chicken mince into the cheese mixture.

- Set the mushrooms on the prepared baking tray.

- Spoon some chicken filling on each mushroom head.

- On the top of each mushroom, sprinkle some breadcrumbs.

- Put in the oven for 15-20 minutes. They should be slightly brown on the top.

- Serve warm.

3.24. Crispy Shrimp

- Total Time: 35mins

- Prep time: 15 mins

- Cooking time: 20 mins

- Serving Size: 4 servings

Ingredients:

1. 1 kg shrimp peeled and deveined.

2. 2 tbsp lemon juice

3. 2 tbsp chicken stock

4. 1 brown onion

5. 1/4 cup parsley leaves

6. 5 cloves garlic chopped.

7. 1/3 cup melted butter, divided.

8. 2 tbsp parmesan cheese

9. ½ cup breadcrumbs

10. 1/2 tsp crushed red pepper flakes

11. ½ tsp pepper

12. Salt to taste

13. 2 lemons cut in wedges.

Instructions:

- First, preheat the oven to 425° F.

- In a bowl, add the shrimp, chicken stock, ginger, lemon juice, melted butter, pepper, and salt. Mix well.

- Assemble the shrimp in a thin layer towards the middle of a butter paper-lined baking dish.

- Mix the leftover melted butter, cheese, breadcrumbs, chili flakes, garlic, and minced parsley in a bowl.

- Top this shrimp mixture with the breadcrumb mixture.

- Bake for 10-12 minutes. The top should be crispy and lightly browned.

- Sprinkle the leftover parsley and lemon juice.

- Serve while warm.

3.25. Potato Cups

- Total Time: 1 hour

- Prep time:20 mins

- Cooking time:40 mins

- Serving Size: 3 servings

Ingredients:

1. 12 baby potatoes

2. 3 green onions chopped.

3. ¼ cup cream

4. 2 tbsp melted butter

5. 2 tbsp sundried tomatoes chopped.

6. ¼ tsp cayenne pepper

7. ½ tsp paprika

8. ½ tsp pepper

9. Salt to taste

Instructions:

- Preheat the oven to 350 °F.

- Wash and dry the potatoes. Split them lengthwise into two.

- Melt some butter and grease on a baking tray.

- Put the potatoes face down on the baking tray and bake for 30 minutes.

- The potatoes should be cooked, and the skin should be intact.

- Cool the potatoes. Now scoop out the cooked potato leaving the peels in a cup shape. Save this for later use.

- Mix the potatoes, peas, green onions, sundried tomatoes, cayenne pepper, and melted butter with a hand blender.

- Add milk and blend till a mashed potato texture is achieved.

- Fill the potato cups with this filling.

- Sprinkle some paprika on the filled cups.

- Bake for 10-15 minutes.

- Serve while warm.

3.26. Chicken Veggie Stuffed Mushroom

- Total Time: 45 mins

- Prep time: 20 mins

- Cooking time: 25 mins

- Serving Size: 2 servings

Ingredients:

1. 5 large mushrooms
2. 1½ cup baby spinach
3. ½ cup onion, chopped.
4. 1 tsp minced garlic
5. 250g chicken sausage
6. ½ cup parmesan cheese
7. ½ cup melted butter.
8. 3/4 cup breadcrumbs
9. 2 tbsp fresh parsley

Instructions:

- First, preheat the oven to 350 °F.
- Cut the mushroom stems and set them aside.
- In a pan, sauté the mushroom stems, red onions, and garlic. Add cut spinach and cook until the flavors are released.
- Take off from the stove and let it cool down.
- When this mixture is cooled down, add the breadcrumbs and 1 tablespoon cheese.
- Clean the heads of mushrooms and remove gills.
- Coat the mushroom heads with melted butter.
- Spoon the mixture to the mushrooms. Arrange the mushrooms in a butter paper-lined baking tray.
- Bake for 20-25 minutes. Take out from the oven.
- Sprinkle cheese and parsley on the mushrooms.
- Bake for 5 minutes more.
- Serve either warm or at room temperature.

3.27. Baked Garbanzo Beans

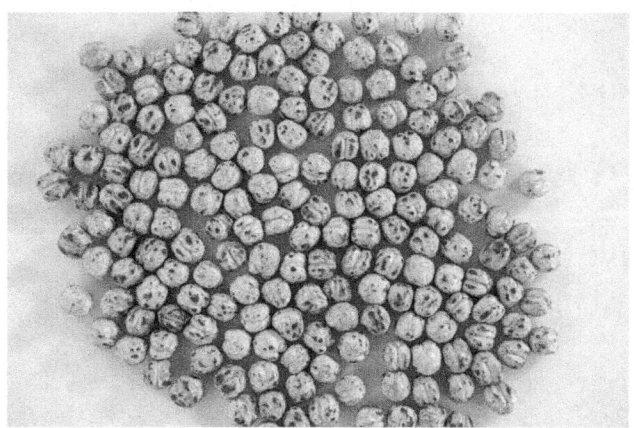

- Total time: 5o mins

- Prep time:5 mins

- Cooking time:45 mins

- Serving Size: 5 servings

Ingredients:

1. 400g chickpeas boiled and drained.

2. 2 tbsp olive oil

3. Coarse salt to taste

Instructions:

- First, preheat the oven to 400 °F.

- Drain and rinse the boiled chickpeas.

- Put them on a baking tray and dry them with a paper towel.

- Drizzle some olive oil on the chickpeas and brush with salt.

- Bake for 40-45 minutes until crispy.

- These can be stored in an airtight container for up to a month.

3.28. Honey Chicken Wings

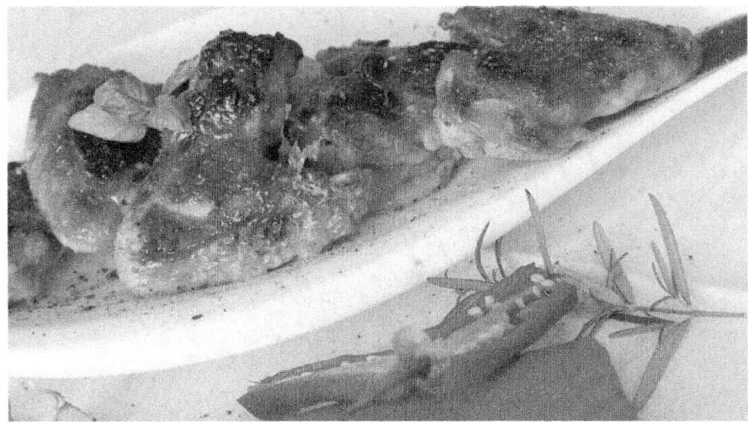

- Total Time: 50 mins

- Prep time: 15mis

- Cooking time: 35 mins

- Serving Size: 6 servings

Ingredients:

1. 2 kg chicken wings

2. 2 tbsp vegetable oil

3. 1/2 cup honey

4. 2 tbsp hot sauce

5. 1 tsp pepper

6. Salt to taste

Instructions:

- Preheat the oven to 425F.

- Prepare a baking tray by lining it with aluminum foil.

- In a wide bowl, put the chicken wings and dry them using a paper towel. To this bowl, add salt, pepper, and oil and coat the wings completely.

- Spread the wings on the baking tray and bake for 25-30 minutes.

- Meanwhile, prepare the honey sauce.

- Add all the ingredients and heat in a saucepan till the mixture becomes a bit thick.

- Take out the wings from the oven. They should be brown and crispy.

- Coat the wings with the honey sauce.

- Bake for an additional 5 minutes.

- Serve hot.

3.29. Fish Fingers

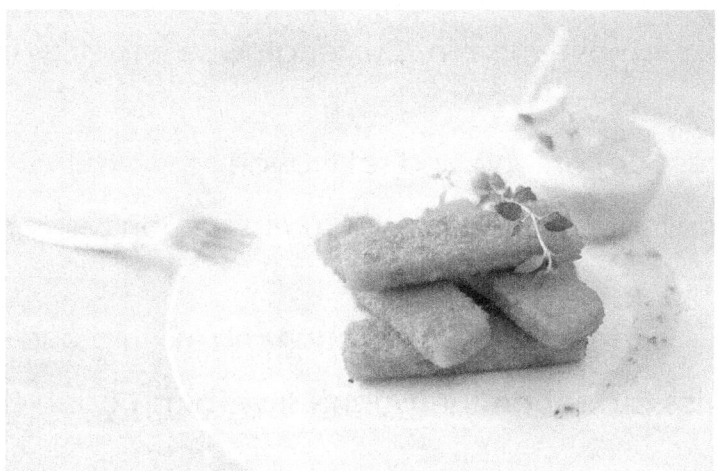

- Total Time: 45 mins

- Prep time: 20 mins

- Cooking time: 25 mins

- Serving Size: 4 servings

Ingredients:

1. 750g white fish

2. 1 egg

3. Salt to taste

4. 1 tsp pepper

5. 1 ½ cup breadcrumbs

6. 4 tbsp plain yogurt

7. 1 ½ tbsp chopped dill pickle

8. 1 tbsp dill pickle juice

9. 1 tbsp lemon juice

10. 1 tsp lemon zest

11. 2 tsp garlic powder

Instructions:

- Preheat the oven to 475°F.

- Prepare a baking tray by lining it with aluminum foil.

- Wash the fish and remove the skin. Cut lengthwise into strips and rub a pinch of salt on each strip.

- On a deep plate, beat an egg and set it aside.

- On another deep plate, mix the breadcrumbs, lemon zest, garlic powder, salt, and pepper.

- Coat each strip with egg and then breadcrumb mixture and set on the baking tray.

- When all the strips are set on the baking tray, brush each strip with olive oil or oil spray.

- Bake for 20-25 minutes, until brown and crispy.

- While the fish is baking, make tartar sauce by combining the yogurt, dill pickle pieces, dill pickle juice, and lemon juice.

- Take out fish from the oven and serve with tartar sauce.

3.30. Cauliflower Fritters

- Total Time: 20 mins

- Prep. Time: 10 mins

- Cooking Time: 10 mins

- Serving Size: 1 serving

Ingredients:

1. 200g cauliflower florets

2. 1 cup Almond flour

3. ½ cup water

4. 1 tsp salt

5. 1 tsp pepper

6. 1 tsp garlic salt

7. Canola oil to deep fry

Instructions:

- In a mixing bowl, mix flour, salt, pepper, and garlic salt.

- Add water to this and make a batter.

- In a deep wok, fill oil and let it heat for 5 mins.

- Next, coat the cauliflower florets in the batter.

- Deep fry each batter in the oil in batches.

- T takes around 1 to 2 mins to fry each floret.

- Take out on a paper towel and remove excess oil.

- Enjoy your snack.

3.31. Fried Peas

- Total Time: 20 mins

- Prep. Time: 5 mins

- Cooking Time: 15 mins

- Serving size: 1 serving

Ingredients:

1. 100g peeled peas

2. 1 small onion chopped.

3. 2 tbsp oil

4. ½ cup water

5. ¼ tsp salt

6. ¼ tsp pepper

7. ¼ tsp cayenne pepper

Instructions:

- In a frying pan, add oil and onions. Fry the onions for 2 mins and add the spices.

- Fry for 1 more minute, and then add the peas.

- Stir fry for 2 mins and then add water.

- Lower the flame and let it simmer till the water is dry.

- Now increase the flame and fry for 2 minutes.

- Serve warm.

3.32. Potato Salad

- Total Time: 20 mins

- Prep. Time: 10 mins

- Cooking Time: 10 mins

- Serving Size: 1 serving

Ingredients:

1. 1 large potato

2. 1 small onion chopped.

3. 3 cherry tomatoes halved.

4. 1 tsp tamarind pulp

5. ½ tsp salt

6. ½ tsp cayenne pepper

Instructions:

- Boil the potato in a large saucepan. Add ¼ tsp salt to the boiling water.

- Peel and dice the boiled potato and put it in a mixing bowl.

- Add all the ingredients and mix well.

- Enjoy the salad.

3.33. Chicken Cheese Balls

- Total Time: 30 minutes

- Prep. Time: 15 mins

- Cooking Time: 15 mins

- Serving Size: 4 servings

Ingredients:

1. 200g boiled chicken

2. 100 g cheddar cheese cut in small cubes.

3. 1 tomato diced and seeds removed.

4. 2 boiled potatoes mashed.

5. 1 tsp salt

6. 1 tsp pepper

7. 1 tsp chopped green chili.

8. Oil to fry

9. 1 egg

10. 1 cup breadcrumbs

11. Oil to shallow fry

Instructions:

- In a large bowl, shred the boiled chicken very finely. Add the mashed potatoes, salt, pepper, and garlic. Then add the green chilis.

- Knead to make a smooth dough.

- Prepare a tray and from 7 to 8 balls. Form the balls such that you place 2 pieces of cheese and two pieces of tomato in the center.

- Now, beat and egg in a small bowl and keep the breadcrumbs in a bowl beside.

- In a wok, heat oil for 2 minutes.

- Coat the chicken ball in egg and then breadcrumbs.

- Shallow fry the chicken ball on all sides.

- Repeat the process with all the chicken balls.

- Put on a paper towel to remove excess oil.

- Serve warm.

3.34. Garden Salad

- Total Time: 10 minutes

- Prep. Time: 10 mins

- Cooking time: N/A

- Serving Size: 2-3 servings

Ingredients:

1. 1 chopped onion

2. 1 chopped carrot

3. 1 chopped capsicum

4. 1 chopped cucumber

5. 50 g chopped lettuce

6. 2 tsp lemon juice

7. 1 tsp olive oil

8. ¼ tsp salt

9. ¼ tsp pepper

Instructions:

- In a large salad bowl, add all ingredients.

- Toss them well.

- Enjoy your fresh and healthy salad.

3.35. Pasta Salad

- Total Time: 20 mins
- Prep. Time: 10 mins
- Cooking Time: 10 mins
- Serving Size: 1 serving

Ingredients:

1. 50 g wheat pasta
2. 1 chopped onion
3. 1 chopped cucumber
4. 1 chopped tomato
5. ½ tsp oregano
6. ¼ tsp salt
7. ½ tsp olive oil

Instructions:

- Boil the pasta and drain it.
- In a large mixing bowl, mix all the ingredients.
- Enjoy your pasta salad.

3.36. Creamy Salad

- Total Time: 15 mins
- Prep. Time: 5 mins
- Cooking Time: 6 to 8 mins
- Serving Size: 1 serving

Ingredients:

1. 50 g wheat pasta
2. 1 tbsp fresh cream

3. 1 tsp mayonnaise

4. 1 diced carrot

5. 50 g peas

6. 1 diced apple

7. ¼ tsp white pepper

8. ¼ tsp garlic powder

Instructions:

- Boil the pasta and drain it.

- Steam the carrots and peas.

- In a large bowl, add the pasta and vegetables.

- Add the apple, pepper and garlic powder and mix thoroughly.

- Mix in the fresh cream and mayonnaise.

- Enjoy your salad.

3.37. Mixed Nuts

- Total Time: 5 mins

- Prep. Time: 5 mins

- Cooking Time: N/A

- Serving Size: 10 servings

Ingredients:

1. ½ cup almonds

2. ½ cup walnuts

3. ½ cup raisins

4. ½ cup peanuts

5. ½ cup pine nuts

Instructions:

- In a large bowl mix all the nuts.
- Transfer in an air-tight container or prepare 10 zip lock snack bags of the nuts mix.
- This can be stored for up to 2 months.

3.38. Cobb Salad

- Total Time: 30 mins
- Prep. Time: 15 mins
- Cooking Time: 15 mins
- Serving Size: 4 servings

Ingredients:

1. 2 chicken breasts
2. ½ head romaine lettuce
3. 1 tomato seeded and chopped.
4. 1 avocado peeled and cubed
5. 2 tbsp chopped chives
6. 3 hardboiled eggs
7. 1 cup crumbled blue cheese.
8. ½ head watercress
9. 1 head iceberg lettuce

Instructions:

- Grill the chicken breasts and slice them into thin strips.
- Chop all the ingredients finely.
- Now take a large salad plate and chill it in the freezer for 30 mins.
- Take out the platter and arrange all the ingredients in neat rows.
- Enjoy your salad.

3.39. Spinach and Onion Fritters

- Total Time: 20 mins

- Prep. Time: 10 mins

- Cooking Time: 10 mins

- Serving Size: 1 serving

Ingredients:

1. 200g fresh spinach chopped.

2. 2 onions chopped.

3. 1 cup Almond flour

4. ½ cup water

5. 1 tsp salt

6. 1 tsp pepper

7. 1 tsp garlic salt

8. Canola oil to deep fry

Instructions:

- In a mixing bowl, mix flour, salt, pepper, and garlic salt.

- Add water to this and make a batter.

- In a deep wok, fill oil and let it heat for 5 mins.

- Add the spinach and onion to the batter and coat them completely.

- Deep fry each batter in the oil in batches.

- T takes around 1 to 2 mins to fry each fritter.

- Take out on a paper towel and remove excess oil.

- Enjoy your snack.

3.40. Potato Fritters

- Total Time: 20 mins

- Prep. Time: 10 mins

- Cooking Time: 10 mins

- Serving Size: 1 serving

Ingredients:

1. 2 p0tatoes

2. 1 cup gram flour

3. ½ cup water

4. 1 tsp salt

5. 1 tsp pepper

6. 1 tsp garlic salt

7. Canola oil to deep fry

Instructions:

- In a mixing bowl, mix flour, salt, pepper, and garlic salt.

- Add water to this and make a batter.

- In a deep wok, fill oil and let it heat for 5 mins.

- Cut thick slices of potatoes.

- Dip the potatoes in the batter and coat them completely.

- Deep fry each batter in the oil in batches.

- T takes around 1 to 2 mins to fry each fritter.

- Take out on a paper towel and remove excess oil.

- Enjoy your snack.

3.41. Raisin Almond Granola

- Total time: 45 mins
- Prep. Time: 10 mins
- Cooking Time: 35 mins
- Serving Size: 10 bars

Ingredients:

1. ¼ cup honey
2. ¼ cup instant oats
3. ¼ cup golden raisins
4. ¼ cup black raisins
5. ¼ cup almonds

Instructions:

- Mix all the ingredients in a mixing bowl.
- Prepare a baking tray with butter paper.
- Preheat oven to 300∘F.
- Spread the mixture in the tray in a layer.
- Bake the tray for 35 mins.
- Take out the tray and let it cool. Cut into small squares.
- This can be stored in an air-tight container.

3.42. Chicken Lettuce Wraps

- Total Time: 15 mins
- Prep. Time: 5 mins
- Cooking Time: 10 mins
- Serving Size: 1 serving

Ingredients:

1. 2 whole iceberg lettuce leaves
2. 100g chicken cubed.
3. 1 tbsp olive oil
4. 1 tbsp mustard
5. 2 tsp lemon juice
6. 15 g chopped cilantro
7. 25 g chopped green onion
8. 1 garlic clove minced
9. 1 small carrot chopped
10. 1 tsp chili flakes

Instructions:

- Chill the lettuce leaves in the freezer for 10 minutes.
- Meanwhile, cook the chicken cubes in 1 tbsp oil for 10-15 mins on low flame.
- Put the cooked chicken in a bowl, mix all the remaining ingredients except for the lettuce leaves.
- On a plate, set the lettuce leaves side by side and spoon the mixture onto the leaves.
- Wrap the lettuce leaves and enjoy your chicken wrap.

Chapter 4.

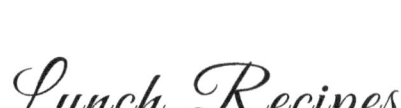

Lunch Recipes

Intermittent fasting is a lifestyle in which sometimes you create a routine where you skip breakfast and break your fast directly with lunch. If you are following that routine, then read on; these recipes will be essential for you.

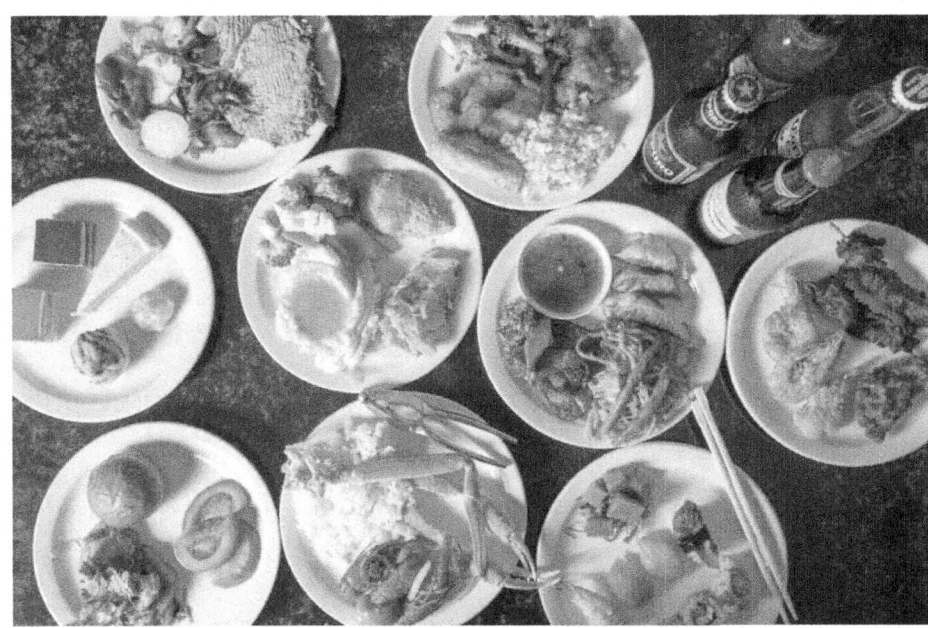

4.1. Chickpea Curry

Chickpeas are a good source of carbohydrates and fiber. This recipe adds a twist of spinach and sweet potato to make it more nutritious and delicious.

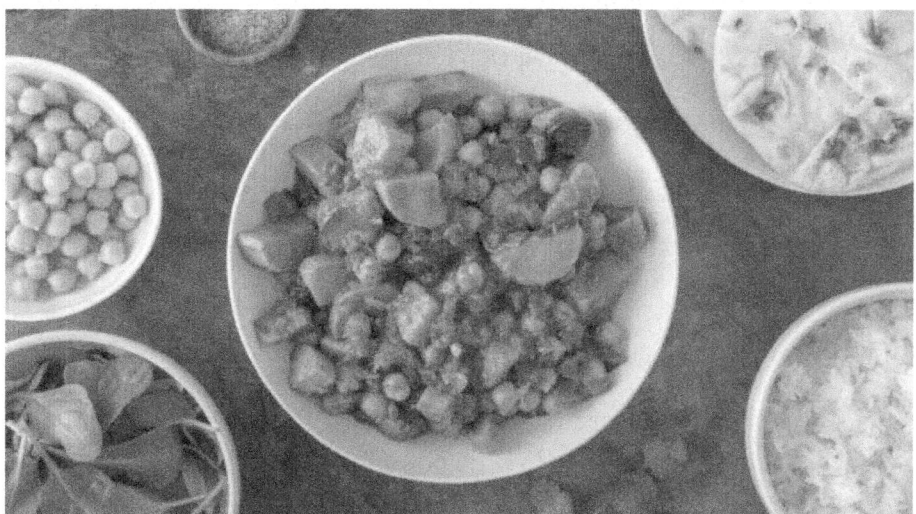

- Total Time: 30 mins

- Prep. Time: 15 mins

- Cook Time: 15 mins

- Serving Size: 2 servings

Ingredients:

1. 2 tbsp vegetable oil

2. ½ red onion thinly sliced.

3. 1 tsp cumin powder

4. ½ tsp cinnamon powder

5. 2 tbsp curry powder

6. 200g canned tomatoes

7. 2 cloves garlic minced.

8. 200g cooked and drained chickpeas

9. 100g spinach chopped.

10. 500 g sweet potato

11. ¼ cup chopped cilantro.

Instructions:

- Peel the sweet potatoes, dice them, and steam them in a steamer for 15minutes.

- In another saucepan, put in the oil and cook the sliced onion for 2 mins.

- Add the garlic, curry powder, cinnamon powder, and cumin powder.

- Cook for 2 mins, so that onion is covered with the spices.

- Add the tomatoes and keep cooking for 5 mins.

- Add the spinach. Keep cooking till the spinach is wilted. It takes about 3 minutes. Keep moving the gravy with a spoon so that it does not burn.

- Next, add the chickpeas and add some water. Cook for 3 more minutes and take it out on a serving dish or bowl.

- Add the cooked sweet potatoes and mix.

- Garnish the dish with fresh cilantro.

- This can be served with white boiled rice or bread.

4.2. Black-eyed beans in a Slow Cooker

If you are a working person, cooking sometimes becomes a difficult chore. In such scenarios, the crockpot comes in handy. This recipe is a bean recipe that you can put in the crockpot in the morning, and when you get back from work, it will be ready.

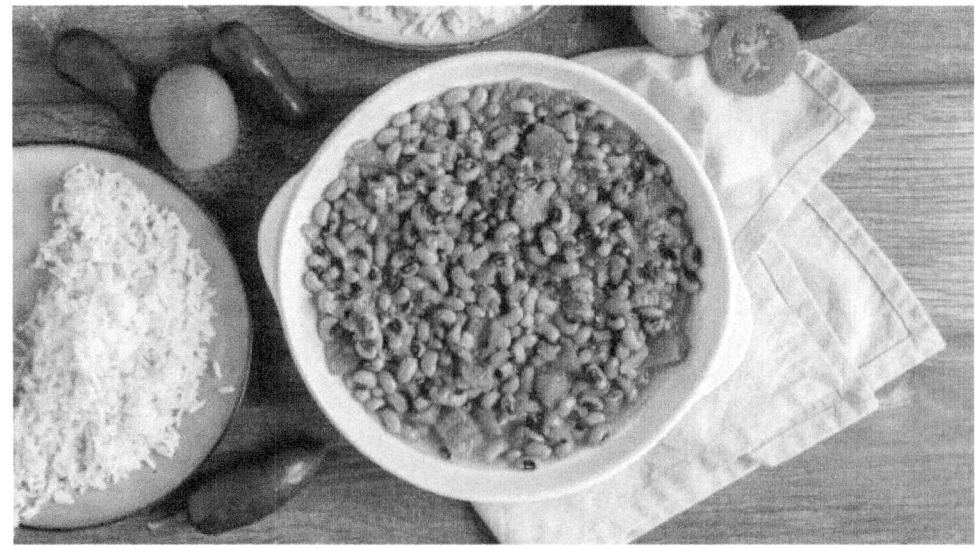

- Total Time: 10 hours

- Prep. Time: 20 mins

- Cooking Time: 9 hours 30 mins

- Serving Size: 2-3 servings

Ingredients:

1. 500g black-eyed beans

2. 200g canned tomatoes.

3. 100g jalapenos

4. 200g chicken breast cut into small cubes.

5. 1 tsp salt

6. 2 cups chicken broth

7. 1 stalk celery chopped.

Instructions:

- Presoak the beans overnight or for at least 4 hours.

- Put in the beans and all ingredients in the crockpot.

- Mix all the ingredients and turn on the crockpot.

- Set the timer to 9 hours.

- After 9 hours, your beans will be ready. Serve with boiled rice or eat as it is.

4.3. Burrito

Bean burritos are a Mexican specialty. Full of protein, dietary fiber, and vitamins. If you prefer a healthier version, always use whole wheat wraps.

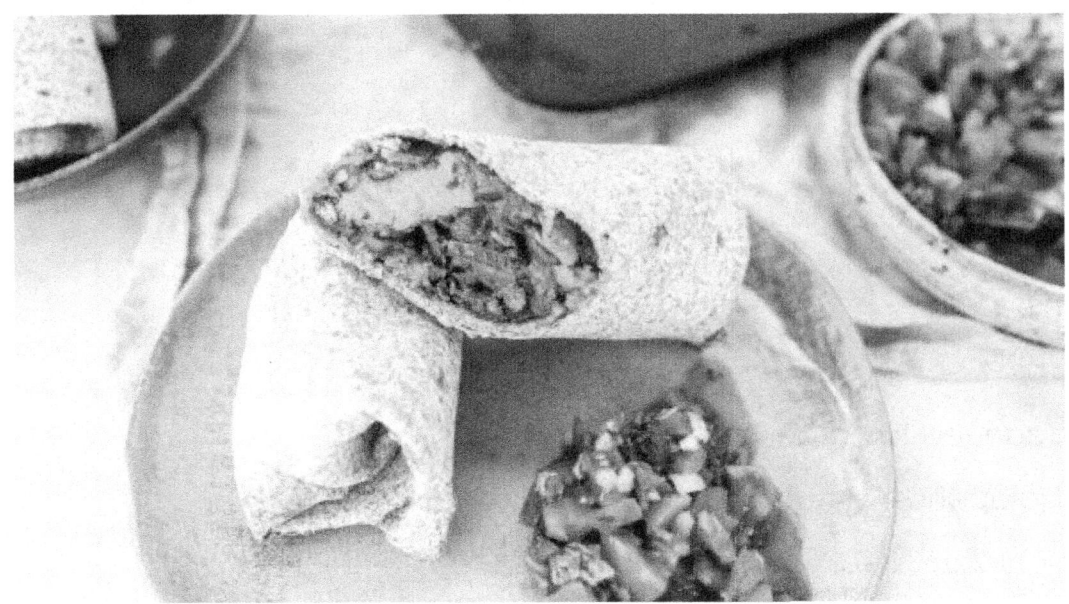

- Total Time: 1 hour

- Prep. Time: 30 mins

- Cooking Time: 30 mins

- Serving Size: 5 servings

Ingredients:

1. 2 cups sweet potatoes cubed.

2. 200g black canned black beans

3. 1 tsp salt

4. 2 small onions chopped.

5. 2 cloves of garlic minced.

6. 1 tsp cumin

7. 2 tsp lemon juice

8. 1/3 cup chopped cilantro.

9. 2 tsp chopped green chilis.

10. 1 tsp coriander powder

11. 2 tbsp olive oil

12. 5 tortilla wraps (10 inch)

Instructions:

- Put the sweet potatoes in a large saucepan, cover with water and add salt. Bring to boil, and then lower the flame. Let it simmer for 10 minutes.

- Preheat the oven at 350∘F. Prepare a baking tray with butter paper.

- Meanwhile, in a frying pan, add oil and onions and sauté for 5 minutes.

- Add the garlic, cumin, coriander powder, green chili, cook for 3 minutes, and then take off the flame.

- When the sweet potato is soft, drain it and put it in the blender. Add the black beans and cilantro.

- When a smooth mixture is formed, take it out in a mixing bowl and add the onion and spices. Mix well.

- Put 3 tablespoons (heaped) of the mixture on the tortilla wraps and fold them snug.

- Place the wraps on the baking tray and bake for 30 minutes.

- Serve hot with salsa sauce.

4.4. Cauliflower Pizza

This pizza recipe is suitable for intermittent fasting, keto diet as well as low carb diet. The pizza crust is made of cauliflower but tastes exactly like the flour crust. Now you can enjoy your yummy pizza without worrying about calories and carbohydrates.

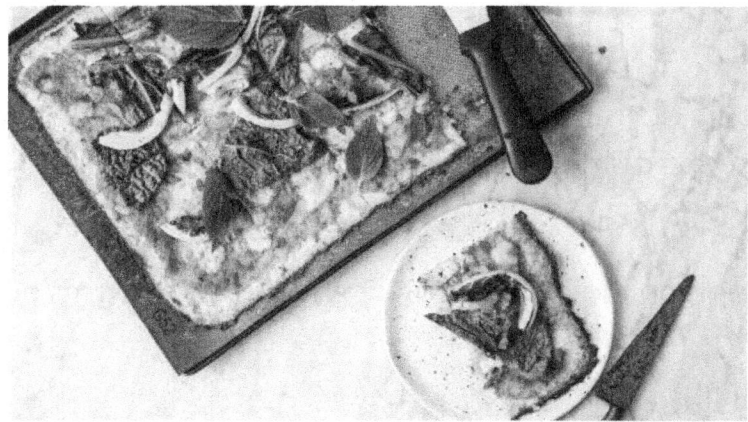

- Total Time: 1 hour

- Prep. Time: 10 mins

- Cooking Time: 50 mins
- Serving Size: 4 servings

Ingredients:

1. 4 cups cauliflower
2. 1 medium egg
3. 1 tsp salt
4. 1 tsp oregano
5. 1 cup goat cheese
6. 4 tbsp pizza sauce
7. Handful basil leaves
8. ½ cup cheddar cheese
9. 1 avocado sliced

Instructions:

- The first step is to make cauliflower rice. In a food processor, add the cauliflower florets on the cup, and turn on the processor. Stop when a rice-like texture is obtained. Repeat the process with the entire amount of cauliflower.
- Now in a large saucepan, add the rice and cover with water. Add salt. Bring to boil, and then turn down the flame. Let it simmer for 10 minutes.
- Strain the cauliflower rice and squeeze out all the water.
- In a mixing bowl, add the rice, egg, oregano, and goat cheese. Kneed all the ingredients to make a smooth dough.
- Preheat the oven at 350°F and prepare a baking tray with butter paper.
- Spread the dough on the baking tray and raise the dough's edges to give the crust effect.
- Bake for 35 minutes.
- Take out the pizza crust and put on the toppings. Spread the pizza sauce, then add the cheese, avocado slices, and basil leaves. You can add toppings of your choice as well.

- Bake for 5 to 10 minutes.

- Serve hot.

4.5. Baked Chicken

This is an oven recipe and simple to follow. There are few ingredients and makes a delicious chicken lunch.

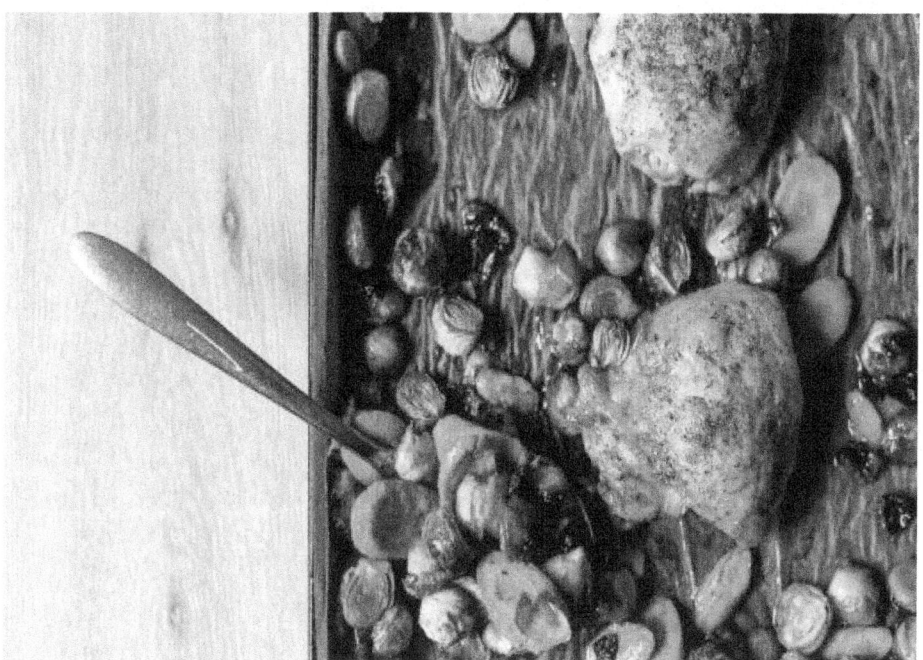

- Total Time: 45 minutes

- Prep. Time: 10 minutes

- Cooking Time: 35 mins

- Serving Size: 4 servings

Ingredients:

1. 4 chicken thighs with skin

2. 3 tbsp olive oil

3. 1 tsp salt

4. 1 tsp pepper

5. 1 tsp oregano

6. 1 tsp thyme

7. 1 cup Brussel sprouts cut in half.

8. 2 cups carrots cut in thick slices.

Instructions:

- Preheat oven to 400°F.

- Prepare a large baking tray with butter paper.

- In a mixing bowl, add the vegetables and drizzle 1 tbsp oil and toss them.

- Add salt, pepper, oregano, and thyme to the vegetables and mix well.

- A small bowl makes a mixture of the remaining oil, salt, pepper, thyme, and oregano. Rub this mixture on the chicken thighs.

- Spread the vegetables on the baking tray and put the chicken thighs over the vegetables.

- Put the tray in the oven for 35 minutes.

- When the chicken is done, serve warm.

4.6. Chicken and Yogurt

This is a simple recipe. It has a few ingredients and gives off aromatic flavors. High in protein and keeps you full for a long period.

- Total time: 40 mins

- Prep. Time: 20 mins

- Cook Time: 20 mins

- Serving Size: 2 servings

Ingredients:

1. 2 boneless chicken breasts

2. 1 cup yogurt

3. 1 tsp salt

4. 1 tsp red chili

5. 1 tsp cumin

6. ½ tsp turmeric

7. ¼ cup oil

Instructions:

- Cut the chicken breasts into small cubes.

- In a mixing bowl, add yogurt, salt, chili, turmeric, and cumin and marinate for chicken.

- Add the chicken cubes to this marinate and ensure that the chicken pieces are covered in this marinate.

- Leave for 20 minutes.

- After 20 minutes, in a large saucepan, pour the oil. Turn on the flame and add the chicken.

- Cook on high flame for 5 minutes and then turn down the flame.

- Cook for 20 to 25 minutes on medium flame, moving the chicken with the spoon at 5 minutes intervals so that the chicken does not stick.

- After 20 mins, cook the chicken at high flame for 2 minutes.

- Take out in a serving plate and serve warm.

4.7. Chicken Pizza

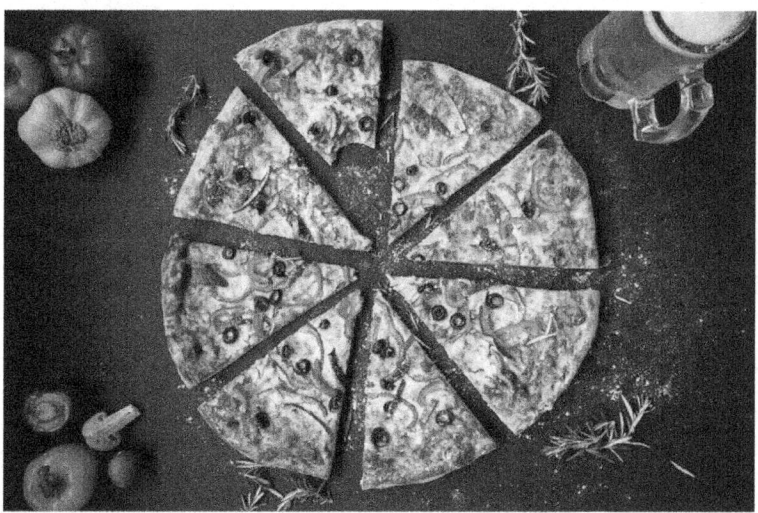

- Total Time: 1 hour 5 mins

- Prep time: 40 mins

- Cooking time: 25 mins
- Serving Size: 4 servings

Ingredients:

1. 1 cup boiled chicken (boneless)
2. 1 cup almond flour
3. 1 egg
4. 1 onion chopped.
5. 2 tomatoes diced.
6. 1 tomato sliced.
7. 1 bell pepper sliced.
8. 2 tbsp sliced olives
9. 100g mozzarella cheese (grated)
10. 100 g cheddar cheese (grated)
11. 2 tsp oil
12. ¼ cup milk
13. 1 tsp instant yeast
14. ½ tsp thyme
15. ½ tsp oregano
16. ½ tsp pepper
17. 1 tsp sugar
18. Salt to taste

Instructions:

- Preheat the oven to 350 °F first.
- By greasing 1 teaspoon of oil, prepare an 8-inch pizza baking dish.
- Create the dough in a bowl by mixing wheat, salt, sugar, egg, milk, yeast, and 2 tablespoons of oil. To produce a smooth dough, knead well. If needed, add water. The dough is supposed to be firm.

- Cover it and keep it in a warm, dry spot for 30 minutes. Let the dough rise.

- Shred the chicken with your hands in a different bowl and season it with salt and pepper.

- Put 2 teaspoons of oil into a saucepan, place the chopped onion and stir for 2 minutes until the onion is clear. Add the diced tomatoes and wait till they are tender. When the tomatoes are tender, turn off the flame and add the oregano and thyme.

- Now examine the dough. It should rise to double. Roll it out on the pizza dish. Pinch the dough at all corners.

- Poke the pizza base at four to five spots with a fork.

- Placed the pizza base in the oven for 5 minutes without topping, which is called blind baking.

- Remove the pizza base. On the base, spread the tomato sauce. Top with the chicken. Distribute it uniformly.

- Now top it with olives, slices of tomato and capsicum. Cover it with cheddar cheese and mozzarella. Distribute it all equally.

- Place in the oven for 20-25 mins to roast.

- Serve hot.

4.8. Vegetarian Pizza

- Total Time: 1 hour
- Prep time: 35 mins
- Cooking time: 25 mins
- Serving Size: 4 servings

Ingredients:

1. 1 cup almond flour
2. 1 egg
3. 1 onion chopped.
4. 1 onion sliced.

5. 2 tomatoes diced.

6. 1 tomato sliced.

7. 1 bell pepper sliced.

8. 2 tbsp sliced olives

9. 5 button mushrooms sliced.

10. 100g mozzarella cheese (grated)

11. 100 g cheddar cheese (grated)

12. 2 tbsp oil

13. ¼ cup milk

14. 1 tsp instant yeast

15. ½ tsp thyme

16. ½ tsp oregano

17. ½ tsp pepper

18. 1 tsp sugar

19. Salt to taste

Instructions:

- First, preheat the oven to 350 °F.

- Prepare an 8inch pizza baking dish by greasing with 1 teaspoon oil.

- In a bowl, prepare the dough by adding flour, salt, sugar, egg, milk, yeast, and two tablespoons of oil. Knead well to make a smooth dough. Add water if required. The dough should be firm.

- Cover it and leave it for 30 minutes in a warm, dry place. Let the dough rise.

- In a saucepan, add two teaspoon oil, put the chopped onion, and stir it for 2 minutes until the onion is transparent. Add the diced tomatoes and wait for them to be soft. When the tomatoes are soft, turn off the flame and add thyme and oregano.

- Now check the dough. If it rises to double, then roll it out the size of the pizza dish. And spread it on the dish. Pinch the dough at all corners to create a nice crust edge.

- With a fork, poke the pizza base at four or five spots.

- Put the pizza base without topping in the oven for 5 minutes. This is called blind baking.

- Take out the pizza base. Spread the tomato sauce on the base. Top it with the chicken. Spread it evenly.

- Now cover with mushrooms, olives, tomato slices, and capsicum. Top it with mozzarella and cheddar cheese. Distribute everything evenly.

- Put in the oven to bake for 20-25 mins.

- Serve warm.

4.9. Beef Mince Lasagna

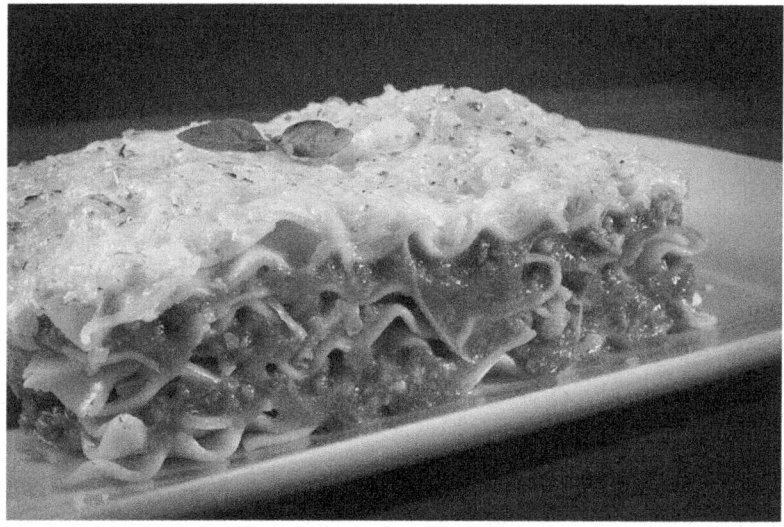

- Total Time: 1 hour 25 mins

- Prep. time: 40 mins

- Cooking time: 45 mins

- Serving Size: 4 servings

Ingredients:

1. 250g beef mince

2. 250g instant lasagna pasta

3. 8 tomatoes diced.

4. 2 onions chopped.

5. 1 carrot grated.

6. 3 tbsp flour

7. 3 tbsp butter

8. 2 cup milk

9. 100g mozzarella cheese

10. 100g cheddar cheese

11. 4 tbsp oil

12. ½ tsp pepper

13. 1 tbsp garlic paste.

14. 1 tbsp ginger paste

15. Salt to taste

Instructions:

- First, preheat the oven to 325 °F.

- Prepare a rectangle-shaped ovenproof dish for baking. Grease it on all sides.

- In a large saucepan, add oil and onions and sauté. When the onions are transparent, add the beef mince and cook for at least 10 minutes. Add ginger paste and garlic paste.

- Now add the diced tomatoes and carrots and let it cook on low flame for 35minutes.

- After 35 minutes, check the beef, it should be ready, and the sauce should be runny. It should not be dry. Take care while cooking that the sauce does not dry.

- In a separate saucepan, make the white sauce. Melt butter and add the flour. Mix it well. Add the milk and keep stirring on low flame. Take care; no lumps are formed. Keep on heating till the milk is half left.

- Add the cheddar cheese and take off the flame. Keep mixing till a smooth sauce is formed.

- Now on the baking dish, spread a layer of beef mince sauce. Then cover with the layer of lasagna pasta. Take care that lasagna sheets do not remain dry. Spread a white sauce layer.

- Again, spread a beef mince layer followed by a lasagna layer and then the white sauce layer. Do the layering in this order till all material is used up.

- Top it with mozzarella cheese spread evenly.

- Bake for 40 minutes. Checking for doneness at regular intervals.

- Serve hot.

4.10. Baked Seabass

- Total Time: 35 mins

- Prep time: 10 minutes

- Cooking time: 25 minutes

- Serving size: 2-3 serving

Ingredients:

1. 750g sea bass

2. ¾ tbsp sesame oil

3. 2 clove garlic sliced.

4. 2 green onions

5. 2 tbsp ginger slices

6. 1 ½ soy sauce

7. ½ tbsp rice vinegar

Instructions

- First, preheat the oven to 400 °F.

- Snip the corners of the spring onions and peel off the rough outer layer (both dark green and stem). Break them into 5-7 cm (approximately 2-3 inch) bits and cut them by the length in half. Slice the ginger into thin strips and peel and chop the garlic into small pieces.

- Cover a baking dish wide enough to accommodate the fish with a sheet of aluminum foil that is large enough to fold the fish together with a little extra. Spread a layer of onion, ginger, and garlic at the bottom of the foil.

- Create two cuts on each side of the sea bass, then put them on top of the onion, garlic, and ginger slices.

- Place in the dish a few more bits of onion, ginger, and garlic, then place the few slices of garlic and ginger into the slits on the side of the fish.

- One onion should still be remaining.

- Combine the soya sauce, rice vinegar, and sesame oil and spread over the fish. To close the package, wrap the fish into the foil and secure it on the edges by folding.

- Bake in the oven for around 25-30 minutes.

- Check for doneness. The fish should be thoroughly done.

- Serve hot, topped with the remaining onion.

4.11. Oven Roasted Chicken

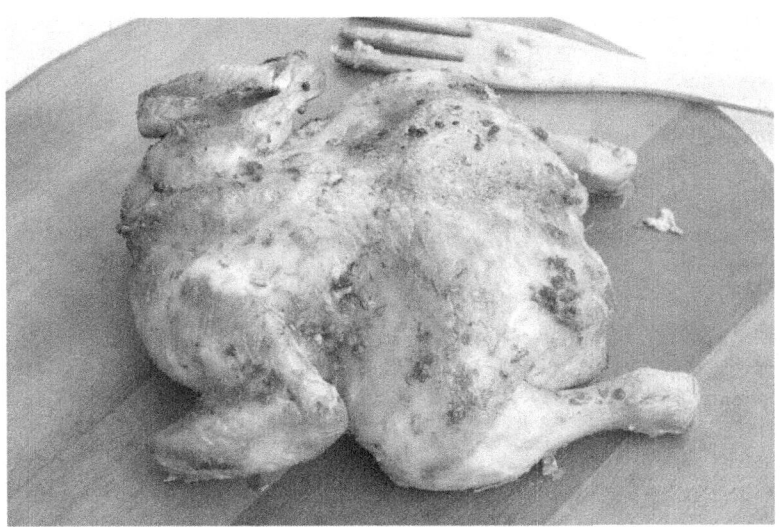

- Total Time: 1 hour 15 mins

- Prep time: 15 minutes

- Cooking time: 1 hour

- Serving size: 4-5 servings

Ingredients:

1. 1 whole chicken

2. 7 garlic cloves sliced.

3. 4 tbsp fresh thyme chopped.

4. 1 lemon zest

5. 50g fresh parsley

6. 5 stems thyme

7. 2 tbsp fresh rosemary chopped.

8. 1 tsp black pepper

9. Salt to taste

Instructions:

- Before anything else, preheat the oven to 400 °F.

- Line a large baking tray with butter-paper.

- Thinly slice 4 cloves of garlic. Mix with fresh chopped rosemary, chopped fresh thyme, and lemon zest in a bow. Rub this mix evenly on the chicken.

- Rub this mix evenly on the chicken.

- Slice the zested lemon into thin circles. Tuck them inside the chicken with parsley and place the leftover cloves of whole garlic and a bunch of fresh thyme inside the chicken.

- Sprinkle the salt and pepper on the chicken.

- Wrap the chicken in aluminum foil.

- Put the chicken in a strong, oven-safe pan and place it in the oven's center rack.

- In the leg's thickest section, insert a temperature probe, and set the temperature to 180 °F.

- Check when the temperature is reached 180°F and insert the thermometer in the other thigh.

- Keep baking again till the other thigh reaches 180°F.

- The temperature will be reached in about an hour.

- Take out of the oven and let it cool for about 10-15 minutes.

- Serve hot.

4.12. Beef Teriyaki

- Total Time: 4 hours 45 mins
- Prep time: 3-4 hours
- Cooking time: 45 minutes
- Serving size: 2-4 servings

Ingredients:

1. 1 ½ kg beef steak
2. 2 tbsp garlic (chopped)
3. 1 cup potato (diced)
4. 1 cup store-bought teriyaki marinade
5. 1 onion sliced.
6. 1 carrot sliced.
7. 2 tbsp olive oil.
8. ½ tsp black pepper

Instructions:

- Cut the beef into strips. Remove as much fat as possible.
- Rub the beef with garlic.
- In a large bowl, mix the potatoes, carrots, onions, and beef. Pour the teriyaki marinade and olive oil. Coat all the ingredients with marinade.
- Leave to marinate for 4 hours.
- Preheat oven for 15 minutes at 350 °F.
- Meanwhile, prepare a baking tray by covering it with aluminum foil.
- Spread all the ingredients of the marinade on the tray in a single layer.
- Bake for 45 minutes.
- Check if the beef is tender.
- Serve warm.

4.13. Peppery Roast Beef

- Total Time: 5 hours 30 mins

- Prep. time: 4 hours

- Cook time: 1 hour 30 minutes.

- Serving size: 12 servings

Ingredients:

1. 3kg beef

2. 2 tbsp coarse pepper

3. ¾ cup horseradish grated.

4. 2 tbsp sugar

5. Salt to taste.

Instructions:

- Obtain a large piece of beef meat without the bone. Tie it to form a loaf shape.

- In a small bowl, mix salt and sugar. Rub the beef with this mixture.

- Line a deep baking dish with aluminum foil and place the beef on it. Cover with cling wrap and chill for 3 hours in the fridge.

- Take out the beef after three hours. Remove the cling wrap.

- In a small bowl, mix salt, pepper, and horseradish. Pat horseradish mixture over the top and sides of beef.

- Bake in the oven for 1 hour to 1 ½ hour.

- Take out of the oven and put on a flat tray.

- Cut into thin slices.

- Save the juices released while baking and pour over the meat slices for flavor.

- Serve warm.

4.14. Baked Pepper and Spinach Pasta

- Total Time: 1 hour

- Prep time: 40 mins

- Cook time: 20 mins.

- Serving size: 4-6 serving

Ingredients:

1. 200g spinach

2. 400g red bell pepper cut into thick strips.

3. 400g penne pasta

4. 500g store-bought tomato pasta sauce

5. 100g goat cheese grated.

6. 30g raisins

7. 2 tbsp olive oil

8. 1 tsp dry thyme

9. 2 onions sliced.

10. 2 garlic cloves chopped.

11. 1 tbsp chili flakes

12. 1 tbsp sugar

Instructions:

- First, preheat the oven to 300 °F.

- Prepare the pasta by cooking it in boiling water for 8 minutes.

- Remove the water and set aside the pasta.

- In a separate frying pan, heat some oil and add the onions. Cook for five minutes till the onions start to soften.

- Add garlic and stir for one minute. After that, add the pepper strips. In the end, add the chili flakes. Cook on a high flame for one minute.

- Next, add tomato sauce, raisins, spinach, thyme, and sugar. Keep stirring and cook for 10 minutes on medium flame.

- Put in the pasta and mix well.

- Next, pour all the pasta into a baking dish.

- Bake the pasta for 25 minutes. The dish will start bubbling.

- Wait for the bubbling to finish. Then serve.

4.15. Baked Fish Fillet

- Total Time: 20 mins

- Prep time: 10 mins

- Cook time: 10 mins.

- Serving size: 4 servings

Ingredients:

1. 4 fillets (medium size) of tilapia fish

2. 3 cloves garlic chopped.

3. ½ cup Parmesan cheese

4. 2 tbsp chopped parsley

5. 2 tbsp freshly squeezed lemon juice

6. 2 tbsp olive oil

7. 1 lemon cut in wedges.

8. ½ tsp cayenne pepper

9. ½ tsp pepper

10. salt to taste

Instructions:

- First, preheat the oven to 400° F.

- Oil a baking dish for baking.

- Wash the fish fillets water and dry with a paper towel.

- Put all the fish fillets in the baking dish.

- In a small bowl, mix garlic, cayenne pepper, salt, olive oil, black pepper, and lemon juice. Pour this over the fish fillets.

- Top the fish fillets with parmesan cheese and fresh parsley.

- Bake for 15 minutes. Check for doneness by using a fork. If the fish easily flakes, it is done.

- Serve hot with fresh lemon slices.

4.16. Simple Cod Fish

- Total Time: 15 mins

- Prep time: 5 mins

- Cooking time: 10 mins

- Serving size: 1-2 servings

Ingredients:

1. 2 cod fish fillets

2. 2 tbsp lemon juice

3. 2 tbsp oil

4. 1 tbsp chopped parsley

5. 2 tbsp lemon juice

6. ½ tsp cayenne pepper

7. Salt to taste

Instructions:

- First, preheat the oven to 400 °F.

- Prepare a baking dish by lining it with butter paper or greasing it with some oil.

- Rinse the fish fillets with cold water and pat dry with a paper towel.

- Put all the fish fillets on the prepared baking dish.

- In a small bowl, add lemon juice, salt, and cayenne pepper. Pour this over the fish and rub a little.

- Bake the fish for 12-15 minutes.

- Check for doneness. Use a fork to check if the fish easily flakes. It means it is done.

- Top with fresh parsley.

- Serve hot.

4.17. Honey Garlic Chicken

- Total Time: 55 mins

- Prep. time: 10 mins

- Cooking time: 45 mins

- Serving size: 4 servings

Ingredients:

1. 1kg chicken thighs

2. 1 tbsp olive oil

3. 2 tbsp honey

4. 2 tbsp garlic paste.

5. 3 tbsp honey

6. 1 tsp cayenne pepper

7. Salt to taste

Instructions:

- First, preheat the oven to 350 °F.

- For baking the chicken thighs, prepare a flat baking pan by greasing it with oil.

- Wash and clean chicken drumsticks. Dry them with a paper towel.

- Make diagonal cuts on the chicken meat. Two cuts on each drumstick. This will make sure that the marinade will impart flavor throughout the chicken.

- Put chicken thighs in a baking pan.

- Rub olive oil on the chicken.

- Next, rub garlic paste on the chicken. Rub some into the slits as well.

- Mix salt and cayenne pepper with honey and pour over the chicken. Rub the honey pic on the chicken and to the slits as well.

- Cover the chicken with aluminum foil. Bake for 30 minutes.

- Take out the chicken, remove the aluminum foil and bake for about 10-15 minutes.

- Wait for the chicken skin to turn golden brown.

- Serve hot.

4.18. Baked Chicken Casserole

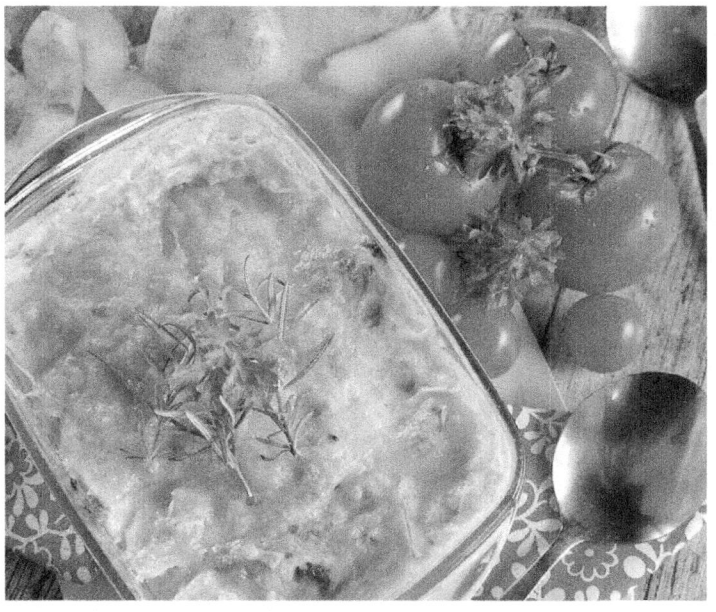

- Total Time: 1 hour 40 mins

- Prep time: 10 mins

- Cooking time: 1 hour 30 mins

- Serving size: 3 servings

Ingredients:

1. 250g boneless chicken cut in cubes.

2. 2 tbsp Ranch dressing

3. ¾ cup shredded cheddar cheese

4. ½ cup heavy whipping cream

5. 5 tbsp unsalted butter cut into small pieces.

6. 1 green onion cut.

7. 2 potatoes peeled and cut into cubes.

8. 1 tsp sugar

9. ½ tsp black pepper

10. Salt or to taste.

Instructions:

- First, preheat the oven to 325 °F.

- Prepare a square baking pan by rubbing it with some butter.

- In a separate bowl, mix sugar, salt, ranch dressing, pepper, and whipping cream. Mix well so that a smooth mixture is formed.

- On the baking pan, form a layer of potatoes. After that, form a single layer of chicken.

- Add a few butter cubes over the chicken and spread with half portion of the cheddar cheese. Top it with green onion.

- Now pour the cream mixture on the top. Cover the casserole with aluminum foil.

- Bake for one hour.

- Take out the casserole. Remove the aluminum foil and bake for 30 more minutes.

- Take out the casserole from the oven. Sprinkle the remaining cheddar cheese and bake again for 10 minutes. This gives a nice brown finish.

- Remove from the oven and serve immediately.

4.19. Baked Tuna and Broccoli Pasta

- Total Time: 1 hour 15 mins

- Prep time: 45 mins

- Cooking time: 30 mins

- Serving size: 6-8 serving

Ingredients:

1. 400g tuna fish shredded by hand.
2. 500g macaroni
3. 250g broccoli chopped.
4. 2 tbsp flour
5. 3 slices sourdough bread
6. 500ml milk
7. 2 red onions are finely chopped.
8. 4 tbsp vinegar
9. 50g butter
10. 2 tbsp mustard
11. 250g cheddar cheese
12. 2 tbsp capers
13. 3 tbsp chopped parsley

Instructions:

- Heat the oven to 300 °F.
- Mix onion and vinegar in a small bowl. Set aside.
- Cook pasta for 8 minutes in boiling water. Drain the water and set pasta aside.
- Put broccoli in a steamer and steam for five minutes.
- Prepare the white sauce. Take a large saucepan, melt the butter. Add the flour slowly and mix. No lumps should be formed. Cook for at least two minutes.
- Turn off the heat and add milk gradually and mix well. Take care that no lumps are formed.
- Turn on the heat and cook on a high flame for two minutes.
- Turn off the heat and add the mustard and cheese and mix till the cheese melts.

- To this sauce, add the pasta and broccoli and half of the parsley. Drain the vinegar from the onion and add the onion to the white sauce.

- Put all of this in a large oven-safe dish.

- Scatter some sourdough pieces on the top of the dish.

- Bake for 30 minutes.

- The dish will be bubbly after taking out of the oven. Wait for it to stop bubbling.

- Serve immediately.

4.20. Baked Turkey Breast

- Total Time: 1 hour 50 mins

- Prep time: 15 mins

- Cooking time: 1 hour 35 minutes

- Serving size: 6-8 servings

Ingredients:

1. 1 turkey breast with skin
2. 3 tbsp flour
3. 1 ½ cup chicken stock
4. ½ cup butter melted.
5. 2 tbsp cream
6. 1 tsp garlic paste.
7. 1 tbsp chopped onion
8. 1 tsp paprika
9. 1 ½ tsp Italian seasoning
10. ½ tsp garlic powder
11. ½ tsp pepper
12. Salt to taste

Instructions:

- Preheat oven to 325 °F.

- Prepare an oven-safe roasting pan for the turkey meat.

- Mix 4 tablespoons of butter, Italian seasoning, garlic powder, salt, pepper, and paprika in a bowl.

- Put the turkey breast on the roasting pan with the skin side up. With your hand, rub the butter mixture on the turkey breast. Reach beneath the turkey skin with your fingers and rub the butter mixture under the turkey skin. Wrap the meat in aluminum foil.

- Pour the remaining butter mixture over the turkey breast and put it to roast for 1 hour.

- Insert a thermometer in the thickest part of the meat. Set it at 165°F.

- When the meat's juices run clear, and the thermometer reaches the 165°F mark, roast for 30 more minutes.

- Take out the turkey breast from the oven and let it cool down for 10-15 minutes.

- Meanwhile, in a saucepan, pour all the clear juices from the turkey roast. Take off all the fat.

- Chop a small onion and put it in the saucepan. Fry it till it is light brown.

- Add the chicken stock and flour. Keep on the heat and mix it till uniform and thick gravy is formed. Remove from flame and add two tablespoons of cream.

- Slice the turkey breast and pour the gravy into the cuts for taste.

- Serve hot.

4.21. Beef Stew

- Total Time: 5 hours 15 mins

- Prep time: 15 mins

- Cook time: 5 hours.

- Serving size: 6 servings

Ingredients:

1. 1 kg beef cubes
2. 3 ½ tbsp. corn flour
3. ½ cup water
4. 1 cup tomato sauce
5. 5 potatoes, chopped.
6. 1 onion, chopped.
7. 8 carrots, chopped.
8. ½ tsp pepper
9. 2 tsp white sugar
10. Salt to taste

Instructions:

- Preheat oven at 225°F.
- In a large oven-safe pot, mix the potatoes, meat, carrots, and onions.
- In a separate bowl, mix tomato sauce, corn flour, salt, sugar, and pepper.
- Put the tomato sauce mixture over the vegetables and meat.
- Cover this mixture with an oven-safe lid.
- Put the pot in the oven and bake for four hours.
- Check for doneness when meat is tender. Take out of the oven.
- Serve hot.

4.22. Baked Okra

- Total Time: 35 mins
- Prep time: 10 mins
- Cook time: 25 mins.
- Serving size: 4 servings

Ingredients:

1. 500g okra
2. ½ tsp garlic powder
3. ¼ tsp ground black pepper
4. 2 tsp olive oil
5. ½ cup cornmeal
6. ½ cup breadcrumbs

Instructions:

- First, preheat an oven to 350 °F.
- Prepare a baking tray, and on the top of the baking tray, place a baking rack. Oil the baking tray and baking rack generously with oil.
- Wash the okra and pat dry. Cut it into ¾ inch pieces.
- Dry the okra by patting it with a paper towel. The drying is especially important. If any moisture is left, the okra can taste soggy rather than crunchy.
- In a large bowl, add garlic powder, pepper, cornmeal, breadcrumbs, and pepper. Add all the cut okra into this mixture and fully coat it with the mixture.
- After coating, place the okra on the prepared baking rack as a single layer.
- It takes 20-25 minutes to make the okra brown and crunchy.
- Check for doneness and serve warm.

4.23. Oven-Baked Veggies with Rice

- Total Time: 1 hour 45 mins
- Prep time: 45 minutes
- Cooking time:1 hour
- Serving size: 8 servings

Ingredients:

1. 2 cups Brown Rice

2. 400g boiled garbanzo beans

3. 400g cooked navy beans

4. 1 eggplant

5. 1 large tomato, chopped.

6. 2 tsp minced garlic

7. 1 cup onion chopped.

8. 4 ½ cup vegetable broth

9. ¾ cup plain yogurt

10. 2 tsp vegetable oil

11. ¼ tsp black pepper

12. ¼ tsp turmeric

13. Salt to taste

Instructions:

- First, preheat the oven to 325 °F.

- Prepare a large casserole dish by lightly greasing it with oil.

- In a separate saucepan, add onion and fry it in oil till it is light brown. Add turmeric, garlic, salt, and pepper. Stir in one or two times. Then add the broth and rice. Lower the flame and let it cook for about 30 minutes. The saucepan should be covered.

- Meanwhile, you can cut the eggplant into ½ inch thick slices. Rub the slices with a little salt on both sides. After 15 minutes, wash them and pat them dry with a paper towel.

- Again, sprinkle some salt on the eggplant slices and drizzle oil on each slice. In a hot pan, cook the eggplant on each side for one minute. Set all the eggplant slices aside on a separate plate.

- Check the rice. If it is cooked and the broth is almost dried, add some yogurt to it and mix. Put this mixture into the already prepared casserole dish.

- Cover the layer of rice with a layer of garbanzo beans.

- The beans are covered by the eggplant, followed by diced fresh tomatoes.

- Bake the casserole for 20 minutes.

- Take out of the oven and serve hot.

4.24. Sweet Salmon

- Total Time: 1 hour

- Prep time: 10 mins

- Cook time: 50 mins.

- Serving size: 4 servings

Ingredients:

1. 300g salmon

2. ¼ cup maple syrup

3. ¼ tsp pepper

4. 2 ½ tbsp soy sauce

5. 2 clove garlic chopped.

6. ½ tsp garlic powder

Instructions:

- Preheat oven to 375 °F.

- Combine the garlic, soy sauce, maple syrup, garlic salt, and pepper in a small bowl.

- Put the fish in an oven-safe glass dish and pour the maple mixture on it. Rub the mixture on the fish so that it is fully coated.

- Put a cling wrap on the dish and marinate the fish for 20 minutes in the fridge. After 20 minutes, turn the fish and cover it again. Let it marinate for 20 minutes.

- Take out the baking dish from the fridge and take off cling wrap.

- Bake it in the oven for 20 minutes.

- Check for doneness with a fork. If a fork easily flakes the fish, it means it is done.

4.25. Baked Shrimp

- Total Time: 45 mins

- Prep time: 30 minutes

- Cooking time: 15 minutes

- Serving size: 6 servings

Ingredients:

1. 1 kg raw shrimp, shelled, deveined, with tails attached.

2. 1 cup butter

3. 1 tbsp fresh lemon juice

4. 2 tbsp mustard

5. 1 ½ tbsp chopped garlic

6. 2 tbsp chopped fresh parsley.

Instructions:

- Preheat oven to 400 °F.

- In a saucepan, mix the mustard, butter, garlic, lemon juice, and parsley. Heat it on medium flame. Let the butter melt. After the butter melts, take the saucepan off the pan.

- Put the shrimp in a high-rimmed baking dish. Put the lemon butter on the shrimp.

- Bake in the oven for 12 -15 minutes. Check for doneness.

- The shrimps should be pink.

- Serve hot.

Chapter 5.

Dinner Recipes

When following intermittent fasting, some people prefer eating an early dinner, and some prefer dinner later in the evening. Whatever suits your body and health requirements should be your choice. This chapter discusses simple and easy recipes for dinner.

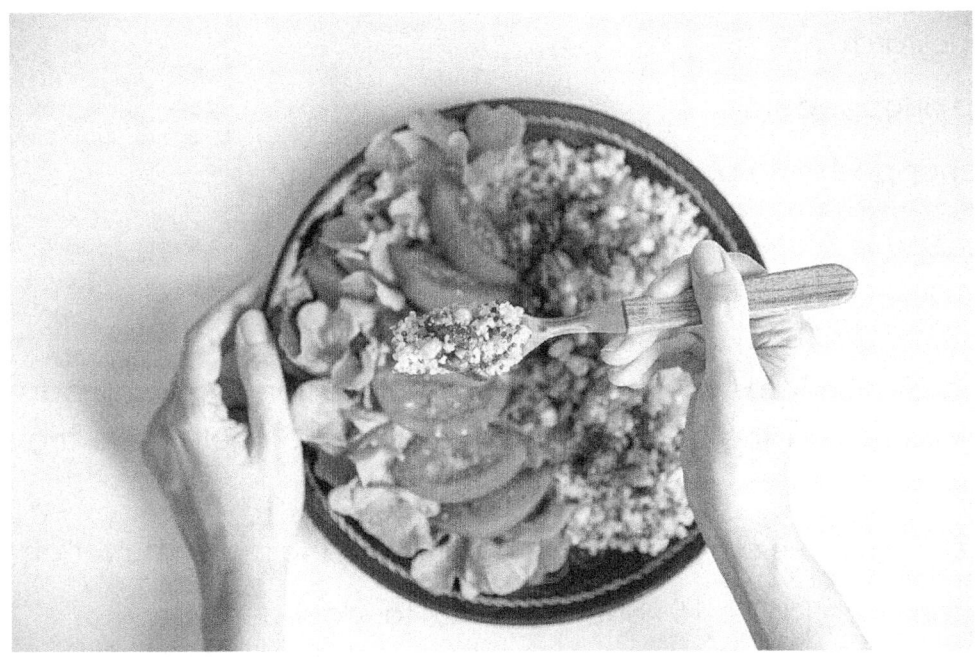

5.1. Beef Chili

Beef is a good source of protein but should be consumed in moderation at 50 plus because it has been linked to heart disease. However, occasionally you can treat yourself with beef.

- Total Time: 45 minutes
- Prep. Time: 10 mins

- Cooking Time: 35 mins
- Serving Size: 2 servings

Ingredients:

1. 200 g beef thinly sliced.
2. 2 tbsp ginger thinly sliced.
3. 5 green chilis sliced longitudinally.
4. ½ tsp salt
5. ½ tsp pepper
6. 2tbsp vinegar
7. 2 tbsp soy sauce
8. 1 tbsp chili sauce
9. 2 tbsp olive oil

Instructions:

- In a wok, add oil and beef slices. Cook for 5 mins on medium flame.
- Add vinegar, soy sauce, chili sauce, salt, and pepper.
- Cook on low flame for 2o minutes.
- Add the ginger and green chili.
- Cook for 5 more minutes.
- Serve warm with boiled rice.

5.2. Broccoli Dal Curry

This is a South Asian dish and is easy to prepare. You can eat it as it is or serve it with boiled rice.

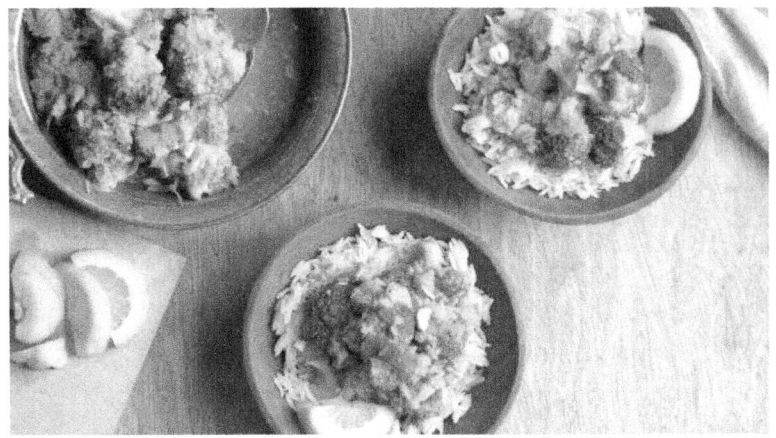

- Total Time: 45 mins
- Prep. Time: 10 mins
- Cooking Time: 35 mins
- Serving Size: 4 servings

Ingredients:

1. 1 cup red lentils
2. 1 medium broccoli
3. 1 tsp salt
4. 1 tsp red chili
5. 1 tsp cumin
6. 1 tsp coriander powder
7. ½ tsp turmeric
8. 1 onion thinly chopped.
9. 4 tbsp flour
10. 2 tbsp cashew nuts coarsely cut.
11. 3 tbsp butter
12. 2 cups chicken broth

13. ¼ cup dried coconut

14. 1 cup water

Instructions:

- Cut the broccoli and steam the florets for 7 minutes, and then plunge in cold water. The strain and keep aside.

- In a medium saucepan, melt the butter and add the onion. Sauté for 3 minutes. Add the salt, chili, cumin, coriander, and turmeric. Cook for one minute, then add the washed lentils and coconut.

- Add the water and chicken broth and bring to boil. Next, lower the flame and cook on low flame for 35 mins.

- Next, please take out a little water from the lentil saucepan and dissolve the flour in it. Put the mixture back in the saucepan and stir.

- Now add the broccoli to the saucepan and cook for 3 mins on high flame.

- Add the cashew nuts and mix.

- Take off from flame and serve with boiled rice.

5.3. Mahi Fish

This is a simple and delicious seafood recipe and suitable for intermittent fasting. This is high protein and high in omega 3 fatty acids, which are good for bone health.

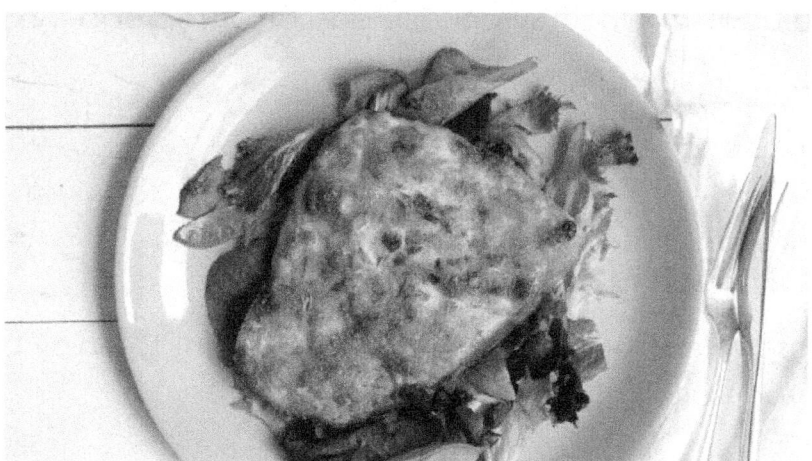

- Total Time: 30 mins

- Prep. Time: 5 mins

- Cooking Time: 25 mins
- Serving Size: 4 servings

Ingredients:

1. 4 fillets of mahi-mahi fish
2. ¼ tsp salt
3. ½ tsp pepper
4. ½ tsp garlic salt
5. 2 tbsp lemon juice
6. 1 cup mayonnaise
7. 1 onion finely chopped.
8. ½ cup breadcrumbs

Instructions:

- Wash the fish fillets with cold water.
- Preheat oven at 425°F.
- Prepare a baking tray with butter paper.
- Put the fish on the butter paper and rub it with garlic salt.
- Next, rub with lemon juice.
- In a separate bowl, mix the mayonnaise and onion. Spread the mixture on the fish.
- Top the fish with breadcrumbs.
- Bake for 25 mins and serve warm.

5.4. Mini Lentil Burgers

Some people choose to eat vegetarian food but still want to enjoy burgers. These lentil burgers are purely vegetarian.

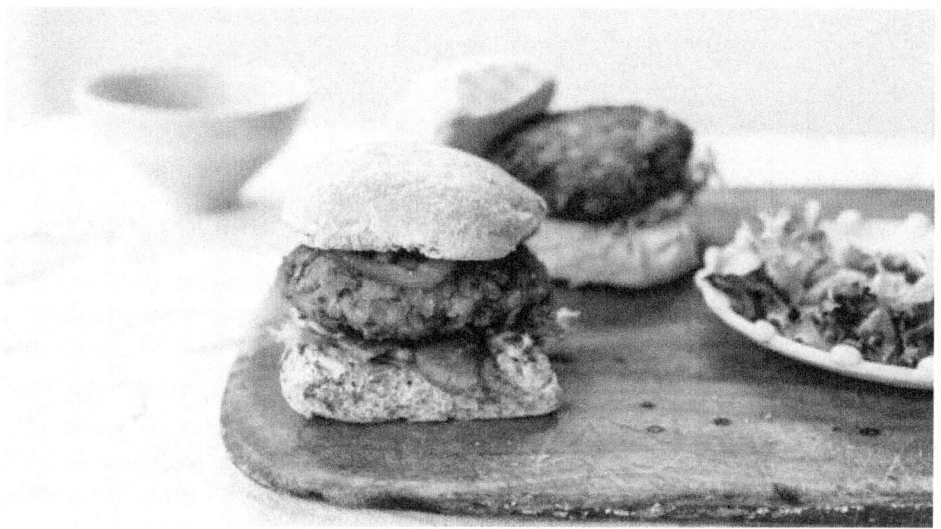

- Total Time: 1 hour

- Prep. Time: 15 mins

- Cooking Time: 45 mins

- Serving Size: 4 servings

Ingredients:

1. 1 cup washed yellow lentils.

2. 2 ½ cup water

3. 1 tsp salt

4. 1 tsp pepper

5. 1 tsp soy sauce

6. ½ cup old-fashioned oats

7. ½ cup breadcrumbs

8. 1 carrot thinly diced.

9. 1 small onion thinly diced.

10. 4 burger buns

11. 2 tbsp olive oil

12. Oil for frying

13. Few lettuces leave.

14.1 tomato sliced.

Instructions:

- In a saucepan, add water, lentils and salt and cook on low flame for 45 minutes. When the water is dried, take it off the flame and put it in a mixing bowl.

- In a frying pan, add oil and onion and carrots. Cook for 3 to 4 mins and add to the lentils.

- Add all the spices and remaining ingredients. Mix with hands, and a smooth dough is formed.

- Make 4 patties and shallow fry or grill on both sides.

- Fill the patties in the burger with salad leaves and tomato slices.

- Serve.

5.5. Fish Tacos

- Total Time: 20 mins

- Prep. Time: 10 mins

- Cooking Time: 30 mins

- Serving Size: 1 serving

Ingredients:

1. 100 g boneless fish
2. 1 small onion sliced.
3. 3 tbsp ranch
4. 1 small tomato sliced.
5. 100 g lettuce chopped.
6. 2 soft shell tacos
7. ½ tsp salt
8. ½ tsp pepper
9. 2 tbsp oil to fry

10. 100 g grated cheese

Instructions:

- In a frying pan, fry fish in oil and add salt and pepper. Cook for 5 minutes and then take out on a plate.

- Now assemble the tocos by putting, lettuce, then fish, then tomatoes and onions.

- Top with grated cheese and fold the toco.

- Enjoy your meal.

5.6. Chicken Toco

- Total Time: 20 mins

- Prep. Time: 10 mins

- Cooking Time: 30 mins

- Serving Size: 1 serving

Ingredients:

1. 100 g boneless chicken breast

2. 1 small onion sliced.

3. 3 tbsp

4. 2 tbsp ranch

5. 1 small tomato sliced.

6. 100 g lettuce chopped.

7. 2 soft shell tacos

8. ½ tsp salt

9. ½ tsp pepper

10. 3 tbsp oil to fry

11. 100 g grated cheese

Instructions:

- Cut the chicken breast into small pieces.

- In a frying pan, fry chicken in oil and add salt and pepper. Cook for 10 minutes and then take out on a plate.

- Now assemble the tocos by putting, lettuce, then fish, then tomatoes and onions.

- Top with grated cheese and fold the toco.

- Enjoy your meal.

5.7. Prawn Tocos

- Total Time: 20 mins

- Prep. Time: 10 mins

- Cooking Time: 30 mins

- Serving Size: 2 servings

Ingredients:

1. 100 g prawns

2. 1 small onion sliced.

3. 3 tbsp ranch

4. 1 small tomato sliced.

5. 100 g lettuce chopped.

6. 2 soft shell tacos

7. ½ tsp salt

8. ½ tsp pepper

9. 3 tbsp oil to fry

10. 100 g grated cheese

Instructions:

- Peel the skin off the prawns and devein them. Wash them with cold water.

- In a frying pan, fry prawns in oil and add salt and pepper. Cook for 3 minutes and then take out on a plate.

- Now assemble the tocos by putting, lettuce, then fish, then tomatoes and onions.

- Top with grated cheese and fold the toco.

- Enjoy your meal.

5.8. Chicken with Rice

- Total Time: 45 minutes

- Prep. Time: 10 mins

- Cooking Time: 35 mins

- Serving Size: 2 servings

Ingredients:

1. 200 g chicken breast thinly sliced.

2. 2 tbsp ginger thinly sliced.

3. 5 green chilis sliced longitudinally.

4. ½ tsp salt

5. ½ tsp pepper

6. 2tbsp vinegar

7. 2 tbsp soy sauce

8. 1 tbsp chili sauce

9. 2 tbsp olive oil

Instructions:

- In a wok, add oil and chicken. Cook for 5 mins on medium flame.

- Add vinegar, soy sauce, chili sauce, salt, and pepper.

- Cook on low flame for 2o minutes.

- Add the ginger and green chili.

- Cook for 5 more minutes.

- Serve warm with boiled rice.

5.9. Mulligatawny Soup

- Total Time: 30 mins

- Prep Time: 10 mins

- Cooking Time: 20 mins

- Serving Size: 2-3 servings

Ingredients:

1. 1 cup yellow lentils

2. 1 chopped carrot

3. 100g peas

4. 1 chopped onion

5. 1 tsp salt

6. 1 tsp pepper

7. 1 tsp cayenne pepper

8. 2 tsp oil

Instructions:

- In a large saucepan, fry the onions in oil for 3 minutes.

- Add the carrots and peas and fry for 3 to 5 mins.

- Now add the washed lentils and spices and add 5 cups of water.

- Let them cook in medium flame for 20 minutes.

- Take out in a bowl and serve warm.

5.10. Tomato Soup

- Total Time: 30 mins

- Prep Time: 10 mins

- Cooking Time: 20 mins

- Serving Size: 2-3 servings

Ingredients:

1. 5 tomatoes

2. ½ cup cream

3. 2 tsp cornflour

4. 2 tsp vinegar

5. ½ tsp salt

6. ½ tsp pepper

7. 2 tsp soy sauce

8. 2 tsp chili sauce

Instructions:

- In a large saucepan, blanch the tomatoes.

- Strain the tomatoes and take off the skins. Puree the tomatoes in a blender.

- Put them back in the saucepan and add 2 cups of water. Add vinegar, soy sauce, chili sauce, salt, and pepper. Cook for 15 minutes on low flame.

- Now take out ¼ cup of soup and dissolve cornflour in it.

- Put it back in the saucepan and stir for 1 minute.

- Take off the soup from the stove and pour in bowls.

- Top with fresh cream and serve.

5.11. Meat Balls

- Total time: 30 mins
- Prep Time: 10 mins
- Cooking Time: 20 mins
- Serving Size: 1 serving

Ingredients:

1. 100 g beef mince
2. ½ tsp salt
3. ½ tsp curry powder
4. 2 tbsp chopped coriander
5. 2 tbsp chopped onion
6. 2 tbsp chopped tomato
7. Oil to fry

Instructions:

- In a large mixing bowl, add the beef. Mix all the ingredients except the oil. Mix well.
- Now make small meatballs. You will be able to make 5 meatballs.
- In a frying pan, heat oil and shallow fry the meatballs on all sides for about 5 to 10 minutes.
- Serve with tomato sauce.

5.12. Chicken Burger

- Total time: 30 mins
- Prep Time: 10 mins
- Cooking Time: 20 mins
- Serving Size: 2 serving

Ingredients:

1. 100 g chicken mince
2. ½ tsp salt
3. ½ tsp curry powder
4. 2 tbsp chopped coriander
5. 2 tbsp chopped onion
6. 2 tbsp chopped tomato
7. Oil to fry
8. 2 burger buns

Instructions:

- In a large mixing bowl, add the chicken mince. Mix all the ingredients except the oil. Mix well.

- Now make two thick burger patties.

- In a frying pan, heat oil and shallow fry the patties on both sides for about 5 to 10 minutes.

- Set them in the burger bun and enjoy with tomato ketchup.

5.13. Beef Burger

- Total time: 30 mins
- Prep Time: 10 mins
- Cooking Time: 20 mins
- Serving Size: 2 serving

Ingredients:

1. 100 g beef mince
2. ½ tsp salt
3. ½ tsp curry powder
4. 2 tbsp chopped coriander

5. 2 tbsp chopped onion

6. 2 tbsp chopped tomato

7. Oil to fry

- For burger

1. 2 burger buns

2. Few lettuces leave.

3. 1 sliced tomato

4. 1 sliced onion

Instructions:

- In a large mixing bowl, add the beef. Mix all the ingredients except the oil. Mix well.

- Now make two thick burger patties.

- In a frying pan, heat oil and shallow fry the patties on both sides for about 5 to 10 minutes.

- Arrange the burger by setting the lettuce on the lower bun and top it with the patty, onion, and tomato slices.

- Serve with tomato sauce.

5.14. Mix Vegetables

- Total Time: 30 mins

- Prep Time: 5 mins

- Cooking Time: 25 mins

- Serving Size: 4 servings

Ingredients:

1. 200g bag of frozen vegetables

2. 2 sliced onions

3. 1 sliced tomato

4. 2 tbsp curry powder

5. 1 tsp salt

6. 1 tsp cumin

7. 3 tbsp canola oil

Instructions:

- Defrost the vegetables and wash them.

- Fry onion in a wide saucepan till brown.

- Add the tomatoes and cook for minutes. Add the spices and keep cooking for further 3 mins.

- Add the vegetables and cook for 5 minutes.

- Add 1 cup water and leave it on medium flame to cook for 10 to 15 minutes.

- When the water is dried, take it off from the stove and serve it with rice.

5.15. Chickpea Gravy

- Total Time: 30 mins

- Prep Time: 5 mins

- Cooking Time: 25 mins

- Serving Size: 4 servings

Ingredients:

1. 200g boiled and drained chickpeas

2. 2 sliced onions

3. 1 sliced tomato

4. 2 tbsp curry powder

5. 1 tsp salt

6. 1 tsp cumin

7. 3 tbsp canola oil

8. ½ cup yogurt

9. 2 tsp chopped green chili.

10. 2 tsp chopped coriander

Instructions:

- Fry onion in a wide saucepan till brown.

- Add the tomatoes and cook for minutes. Add the spices and keep cooking for further 3 mins.

- Add the yogurt and cook for 5 minutes while stirring.

- Add the chickpeas and cook for 5 minutes.

- Add 1 cup water and leave it on medium flame to cook for 10 to 15 minutes.

- When the water is dried, take off from the stove.

- Garnish with green chilis and coriander.

5.16. Ginger Chicken

- Total Time: 30 mins

- Prep Time: 5 mins

- Cooking Time: 25 mins

- Serving Size: 3 servings

Ingredients:

1. 200g cubed chicken

2. 2 sliced onions

3. 1 sliced tomato

4. 2 tbsp curry powder

5. 1 tsp salt

6. 1 tsp cumin

7. 3 tbsp canola oil

8. ½ cup yogurt

9. 2 tbsp ginger slices

10. 1 tbsp ginger paste

11. 1 tbsp garlic paste.

12. 2 tsp chopped green chili.

13. 2 tsp chopped coriander

Instructions:

- Fry onion in a wide saucepan till brown.

- Add the ginger and garlic paste and cook for 1 minute.

- Add the tomatoes and cook for minutes. Add the spices and keep cooking for further 3 mins.

- Add the chicken cubes and cook for 5 minutes.

- Add the yogurt and cook for 5 minutes while stirring.

- Add 1 cup water and leave it on medium flame to cook for 10 to 15 minutes.

- When the water is dried, take off from the stove.

- Garnish with ginger slices, green chilis and coriander.

- Serve with rice.

5.17. Corn Soup

- Total Time: 30 mins

- Prep Time: 10 mins

- Cooking Time: 20 mins

- Serving Size: 2-3 servings

Ingredients:

1. 2 cup corn

2. ½ cup cream

3. 2 tsp vinegar

4. ½ tsp salt

5. ½ tsp pepper

6. 2 tsp soy sauce

7. 2 tsp chili sauce

Instructions:

- In a large saucepan, boil the corn for 5 mins in boiling water and then drain.

- Puree half the corns in a blender.

- Put the puree and remaining corns back in the saucepan and add 2 cups of water. Add vinegar, soy sauce, chili sauce, salt, and pepper. Cook for 15 minutes on low flame.

- Turn off the stove and pour soup into bowls.

- Serve with fresh cream.

5.18. Tilapia with Parmesan

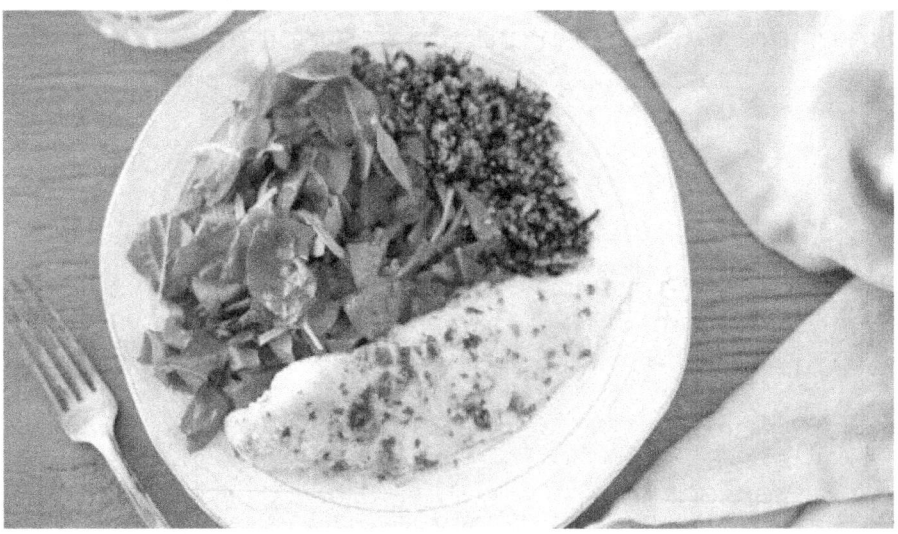

- Total time: 30 mins

- Prep. Time: 5 mins

- Cooking Time: 25 mins

- Serving Size: 4 servings

Ingredients:

1. 500g tilapia fillets
2. 4 tbsp melted butter
3. 3 tbsp mayonnaise
4. ½ cup parmesan cheese
5. 3 tbsp chopped spring onion
6. ¼ tsp salt
7. 3 tbsp lemon juice
8. 1 tbsp dried basil

Instructions:

- Preheat oven to 350°F.
- Line a baking dish with butter paper.
- Wash the fish fillets with cold water and pat dry.
- Set them on the baking dish and rub them with lemon juice.
- Bake for 20 minutes.
- In a separate bowl, make a cheese mix by mixing all the remaining ingredients.
- Take out the fish from the oven and spread the fish with the cheese mix.
- Bake for another 5 minutes.
- Serve while hot.

5.19. Chicken with Avocado

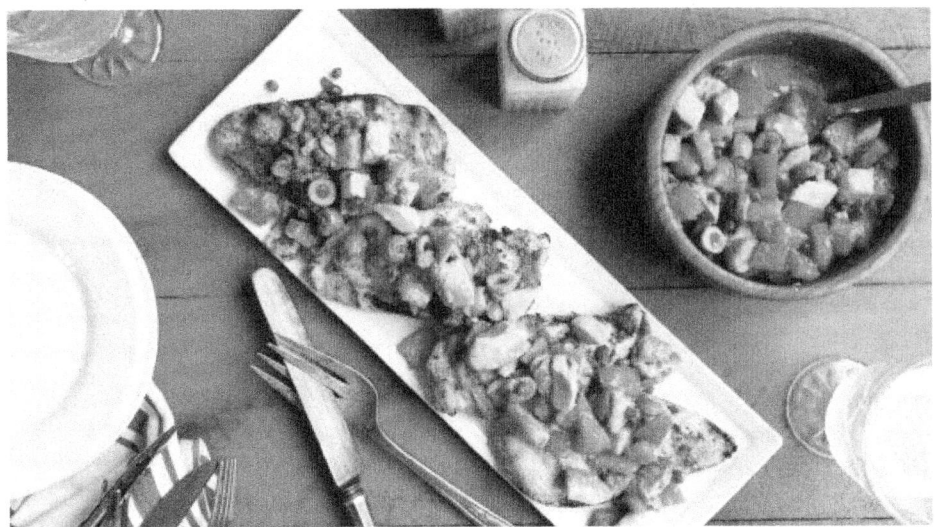

- Total Time: 1 hour
- Prep. Time: 40 mins
- Cooking Time: 2o mins
- Serving Size: 2 servings

Ingredients:

1. 2 boneless chicken breasts
2. 5 tbsp lemon juice
3. 3 tbsp olive oil
4. 1 tsp lemon zest
5. 1 tsp salt
6. ½ tsp ground pepper
7. 1 clove garlic chopped.
8. 1 tomato chopped.
9. 1 ripe avocado cubed
10. 5 green stuffed olives sliced.
11. 2 garlic cloves roasted and mashed.
12. 2 tbsp basil leaves chopped.

Instructions:

- Cut both the chicken fillets in half. Prepare a marinade for chicken in a zip lock bag.

- The marinade is made of olive oil, lemon juice, lemon zest, pepper, salt, minced garlic. Mix all these ingredients in a zip lock bag and put them in the chicken fillets.

- Refrigerate for 30 mins.

- Meanwhile, create an avocado salad by mixing the avocadoes, olives, roasted garlic, tomato, and basil leaves. Set this aside.

- Take out the chicken from marinating and discard the liquid.

- Grill the chicken breasts on medium flame, around seven minutes on both sides.

- Serve with the avocado salad.

5.20. Chicken Salad

- Total Time: 20 mins

- Prep. Time: 10 mins

- Cooking Time: 10 mins

- Serving Size: 2 servings

Ingredients:

1. 1 boneless chicken breast

2. 50 g lettuce chopped.

3. 50 g cabbage chopped.

4. 1 small carrot chopped.

5. ¼ tsp salt

6. ¼ tsp pepper

7. 3 tbsp mayonnaise

8. 4 slices brown bread

Instructions:

- Boil the chicken breast. Remove the water and shred the chicken.

- In a large bowl, mix all the ingredients to make a spread.

- Toast the brown bread and spread the mixture.

- Make a sandwich and enjoy.

5.21. Avocado Quesadillas

- Total Time: 20 mins

- Prep Time: 10 mins

- Cooking Time: 10 mins

- Serving Size: 1 serving

Ingredients:

1. 4 flour tortillas

2. ½ cup jack cheese

3. 1 ripe avocado

4. 1 chopped onion

5. 1 chopped tomato (seeds removed)

6. 2 tsp lemon juice

7. ¼ cup sour cream

8. 1 tbsp chopped coriander

9. ¼ tsp salt

10. ¼ tsp pepper

Instructions:

- On a baking sheet, put the tortillas and bake for 5 mins on a 200∘F setting.

- Next, take out the tortillas and spread the cheese on 2 tortillas and bake for 5 more minutes.

- Meanwhile, mix the sour cream with coriander, salt and pepper and make a smooth spread.

- Apply this spread to the remaining tortillas.

- In another bowl, mix the avocadoes, tomatoes, onion, and lemon juice. Spread this mixture over the sour cream.

- Take out the tortillas from the oven and put them on top of the other two tacos with the cheese size down.

- Cut the tortillas in a wedge shape.

- Enjoy your meal.

5.22. Grilled Salmon

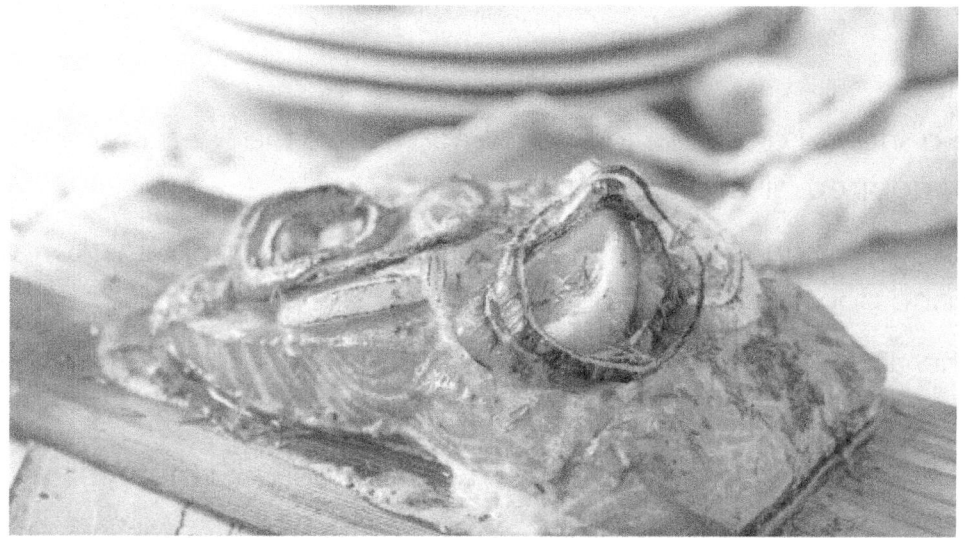

- Total time: 1 hour

- Prep. Time: 40 mins

- Cooking Time: 20 mins

- Serving Size: 4 servings

Ingredients:

1. 750 g salmon fish fillets

2. 2 tbsp dill

3. ½ tsp pepper

4. ½ tsp salt

5. ½ tsp garlic powder

6. ¼ cup brown sugar

7. 1 chicken cube

8. 3 tbsp oil

9. 3 tbsp water

10. 4 tbsp soy sauce

11. 4 tbsp chopped green onion.

12. 1 sliced lemon

13. 2 slices onion rings

Instructions:

- Prepare a shallow glass dish for the salmon. Place the filters in the dish and sprinkle with salt, pepper, dill, and garlic powder.

- Next, mix the green onions with oil, sugar, soy sauce and chicken cube. Make a mixture and pour over the salmon.

- Cover the dish with plastic wrap and put it in the refrigerator. Take out after 20 mins and remove the plastic and turn the fish pieces.

- Again, cover with wrap and put in the refrigerator for 20 more mins.

- Take out the fish and drain the marinade. Place on the grill and top with lemon and onion.

- Keep on medium flame and cover the fish. Cover and cook for 15 minutes.

- Serve warm.

5.23. Chicken Broccoli Dinner

- Total Time: 30 mins

- Prep. Time: 10 mins

- Cook Time: 25 mins

- Serving Size: 1 serving

Ingredients:

1. 1 chicken leg piece with skin
2. ¼ tsp oregano
3. ¼ tsp salt
4. ¼ tsp cumin
5. ¼ tsp garlic powder
6. 50g broccoli florets
7. 1 tbsp olive oil

5.24. Chicken and Mangos Salsa

- Total Time: 15 mins
- Prep. Time: 5 mins
- Cooking Time: 12 mins
- Serving Size: 1 serving

Ingredients:

1. 1 chicken breast
2. 1 tsp cayenne pepper
3. ¼ tsp salt
4. ¼ tap pepper
5. ½ tsp paprika
6. 2 tbsp olive oil
7. 100 g mango cubes
8. 1 small onion sliced
9. 1 tbsp chopped cilantro
10. 1 tbsp lime juice

Instructions:

- Rub the chicken with cayenne pepper, paprika, salt, and pepper.

- In a frying pan, heat olive oil and cook the chicken on a medium flame for 6 mins on each side.

- Take off from the flame and let the chicken rest.

- In a small bowl, mix the mango cubes with onions, cilantro, and lime juice. Toss and make mango salsa.

- Top the chicken with mango salsa and enjoy your meal.

5.25. Chicken with Bok Choy

- Total Time: 35 mins

- Prep. Time: 5 mins

- Cooking Time: 30 mins

- Serving Size: 1 serving

Ingredients:

1. 1 chicken leg piece with skin

2. ½ tsp salt

3. ¼ tsp pepper

4. ½ tsp paprika

5. ½ tsp cayenne

6. 100 g bok choy washed and trimmed

7. 2 tsp sesame oil

8. 1 tbsp green onion chopped

Instructions:

- Preheat oven at 450°F. Prepare a baking dish and line with butter paper.

- Rub the chicken with salt, pepper, cayenne pepper, and paprika. Please put it on a baking tray and bake for 25 mins.

- After 25 mins take out the chicken and let it rest for 5 to 7 mins.

- In a frying pan, heat the sesame oil and stir fry the bok choy and chopped onion.

- Please put it on a serving plate and put the chicken on it, and serve.

5.26. Chicken Curry

- Total Time: 20 mins

- Prep. Time: 5 mins

- Cooking Time: 15 mins

- Serving Size: 2 servings

Ingredients:

1. 1 chicken breast
2. 1 tsp chili powder
3. ½ tsp salt
4. ¼ tsp turmeric
5. ½ tsp curry powder
6. ¼ tsp allspice
7. 30 g sliced bell pepper (red)
8. 30 g sliced bell pepper (green)
9. 30 g chopped green onion
10. 1 cup coconut milk
11. 1 lime cut in half
12. 2 tsp olive oil

Instructions:

- Rub the chicken breast with salt, chili powder, turmeric, curry powder and allspice.

- In a frying pan, heat the olive oil and cook the chicken for 6 minutes each on both sides. Take it out on a plate and cut it into slices.

- In a separate saucepan, cook the bell peppers and green onion for 1 minute and add coconut milk. Simmer for 7 minutes and squeeze half lime in the saucepan and cook for 2 mins.

- Pour the coconut gravy on the cooked chicken and serve with the remaining piece of lime.

Chapter 6.

Desserts

Most of us have a sweet tooth and cannot resist sweets and desserts. However, when you follow the intermittent fasting lifestyle, it is recommended to keep your sugar content in check. In this chapter, you will find delicious dessert recipes that you can make and enjoy guilt-free while intermittent fasting.

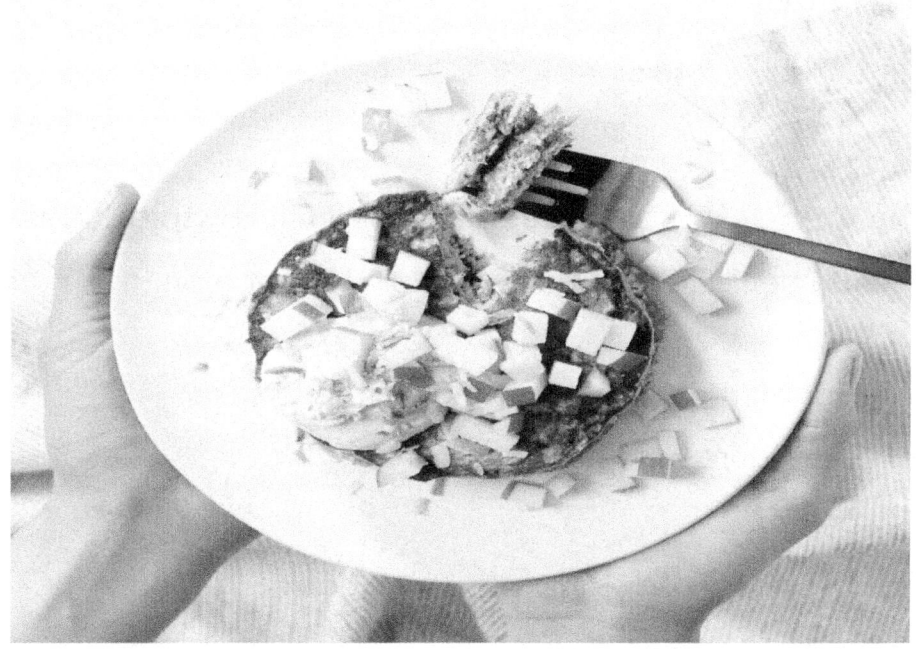

6.1. Vanilla Cherry Pudding

Here is an amazing recipe that is low in sugar and high in fiber, and tastes to curb your craving for sweets.

- Total Time: 45 mins
- Prep Time: 10 mins
- Cooking Time: 35 mins

- Serving Size: 4 servings

Ingredients:

1. 100 g cherries deseeded.
2. 1 pack sugar-free vanilla pudding mix
3. 1 tsp cinnamon powder
4. ½ tsp nutmeg
5. ¼ cup almond milk
6. ½ cup Splenda sugar
7. 1 cup old-fashioned oats
8. 1 tsp vanilla extract
9. 1 cup Greek yogurt

Instructions:

- Preheat the oven at 325°F and prepare a square tin by spraying it with oil.
- Next, put in the berries and mix milk, pudding, cinnamon, and nutmeg. Prepare a mixture.
- In a separate bowl mix all the remaining ingredients.
- Top the cherry mixture with the oat mixture.
- Bake for 30 to 35 mins.
- When baked, take out of the oven and let it cool.
- Put in refrigerator and serve chilled.

6.2. Coconut Muffins

These yummy muffins can be used as a dessert and a breakfast meal if you prefer something sweet in the morning.

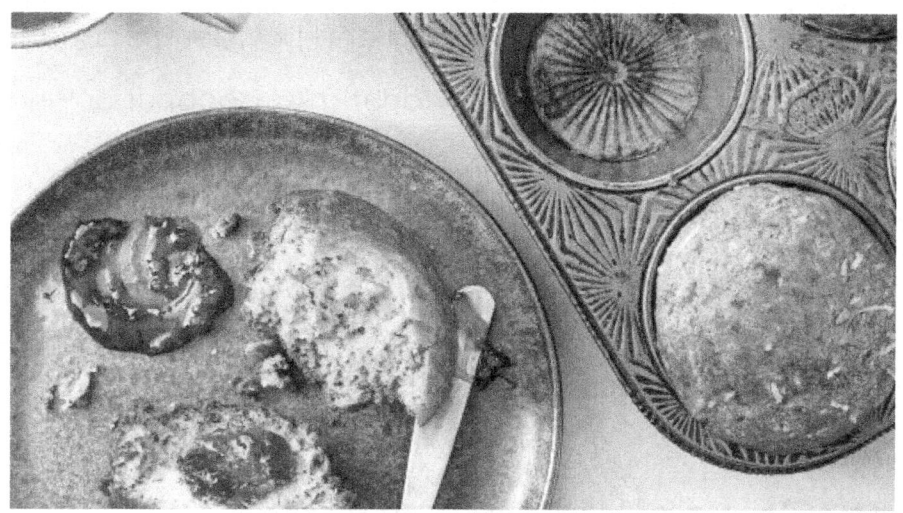

- Total Time: 45 mins

- Prep. Time: 10 mins

- Cooking Time: 25 mins

- Serving Size: 12 servings

Ingredients:

1. 1 cup flour

2. 1 cup sugar

3. ½ tsp salt

4. 2 ripe bananas mashed.

5. 1 cup dried shredded coconut

6. 2 tsp baking soda

7. 1 tsp baking powder

8. 1 tsp vanilla extract

9. 1 ½ cup fermented coconut milk

10. ¼ cup coconut oil

Instructions:

- Preheat the oven to 350°F.

- Prepare a muffin tray of 12 by lining with cupcake sheets or spray them with oil.

- In a bowl, mix the flour, sugar, baking soda and powder, coconut, and coarse salt.

- To a separate bowl, add bananas, coconut milk, coconut oil and vanilla extract. Make a smooth mixture.

- To this smooth mixture, add the dry ingredient mix and mix till a smooth batter is formed.

- Scoop the batter in the baking tray and bake for 30 minutes.

- After making it, the muffins cool for 15 minutes before serving.

6.3. Banana Chocolate Ice-cream

Everyone craves ice cream once in a while. But the ice creams available in the market are full of sugar and artificial flavors. This is the easiest two-ingredient ice cream recipe that will give you the flavor of ice cream without any guilt.

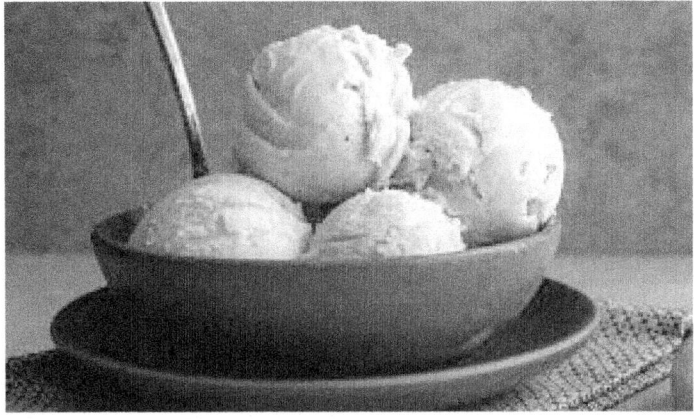

- Total Time: 4 hours

- Prep Time: 3 hours 30 mins

- Cooking Time: N/A

- Serving Size: 1 serving

Ingredients:

1. 2 ripe bananas

2. 2 tbsp chocolate chips

Instructions:

- Peel and slice 2 ripe bananas and store in zip lock bag in a freezer for 3 hours.

- Take out from the freezer and add to a food processor and start pulsing at the highest speed.

- You will see after 3 to 4 mins the pieces will start to form chunks.

- Next, open the processor and scrape the bananas from the corners.

- Again, start pulsing, and you will see the banana will form oatmeal consistency.

- Again, scrape the banana from the corners.

- Keep pulsing, and you will see a creamy texture starts forming. At this point, add the chocolate chips and keep blending.

- Blend for 2 more minutes and scoop the ice cream.

- Enjoy your 2-ingredient ice cream.

6.4. Peanut Butter Cookies

Cookies can be a dessert as well as can be consumed with milk during snack time. This is a simple peanut butter cookie recipe that does not use flour to consume it guilt-free and will not give you an insulin spike.

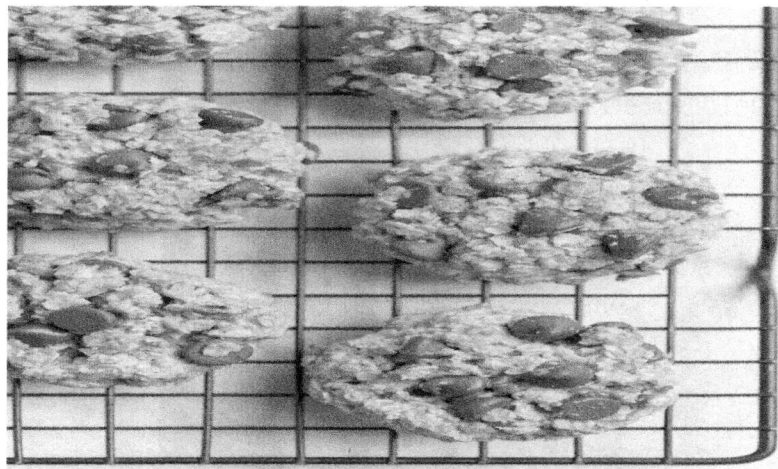

- Total Time: 35 mins

- Prep Time: 5 mins

- Cooking Time: 30 mins

- Serving Size: 2-3 servings

Ingredients:

1. 2 ripe bananas
2. ½ cup instant oats
3. 2 tbsp chocolate chips
4. 2 tbsp peanut butter

Instructions:

- Mash the peeled bananas in a mixing bowl.
- Add the instant oats, peanut butter, and chocolate chips.
- Make a batter.
- Preheat the oven at 325°F.
- Line a cookie tray with butter paper.
- Scoop the batter onto the tray at a 1-inch distance.
- Bake for 30 minutes.
- Let the cookies cool before eating.

6.5. Oatmeal Muffins

This is a healthy twist to the muffins. We use almond flour instead of wheat flour and use a banana instead of sugar for sweetness.

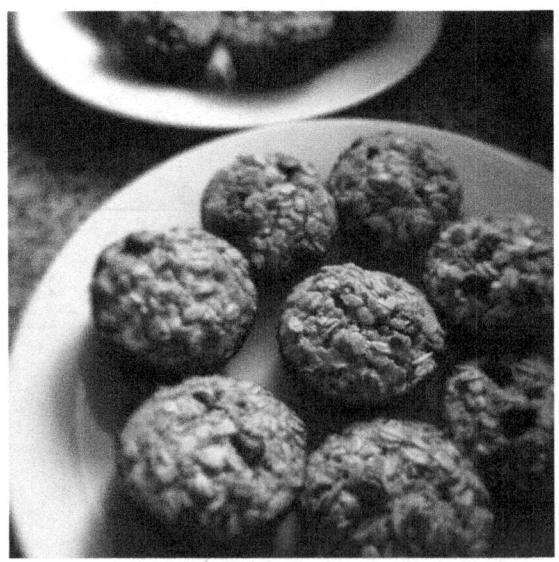

- Total Time: 45 mins

- Prep. Time: 15 mins

- Cooking Time: 30 mins

- Serving Size: 4 servings

Ingredients:

1. 1 cup almond flour

2. 1 ripe banana

3. ¼ cup chocolate chips

4. 1 egg

5. ¾ cup milk

6. 1 tsp baking soda

7. 4 tbsp butter

Instructions:

- Preheat oven at 325°F.

- Prepare a muffin tray by brushing it lightly with olive oil.

- In a mixing bowl whisk the egg and mash the banana in it. Make a mixture and add milk. Further mix well.

- Now fold in the almond flour and chocolate chips.

- When a batter is formed, scoop it into the muffin tray.

- Bake for 30 minutes.

- Please take out the muffins from the oven and let them cool for 10 minutes, and then enjoy.

6.6. Banana Bread

This is an easy recipe that used walnut flour for this recipe.

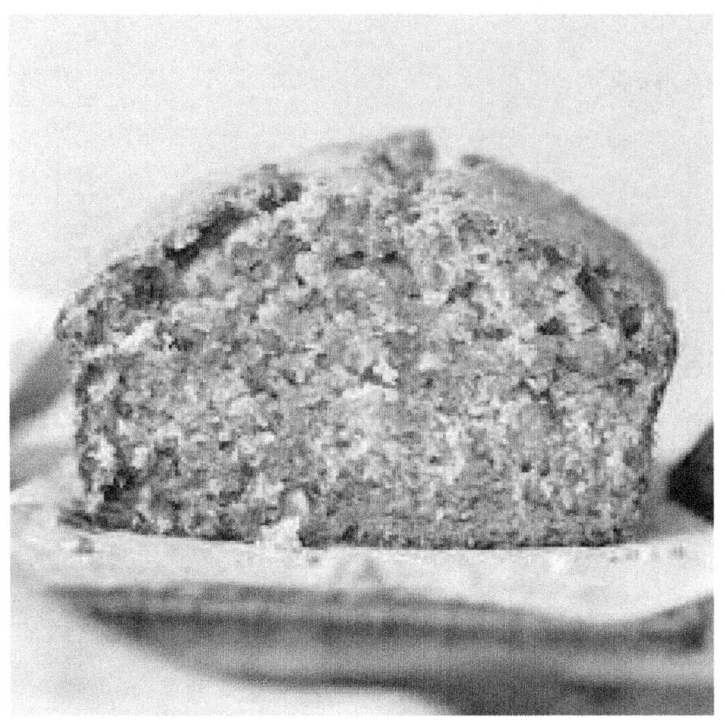

- Total Time: 45 minutes
- Prep. Time: 10 mins
- Cooking Time: 35 mins
- Serving Size: 3 servings

Ingredients:

1. 2 bananas
2. ¾ cup chopped walnuts.
3. 1 cup walnut flour
4. 1 tsp baking soda
5. ½ cup butter
6. 2 eggs
7. 1 tsp vanilla essence
8. ½ cup milk

Instructions:

- Preheat oven at 325°F and prepare a loaf pan by brushing its corners with olive oil.

- In a mixing bowl whisk the eggs.

- Mash the bananas in the eggs and make a mixture.

- Add all the remaining ingredients into the mixing bowl.

- Use a wooden spoon to mix the batter and make a silky mixture.

- Pour the batter into the loaf pan and bake for 35 mins.

- Serve with fresh cream or banana ice cream.

6.7. Blue Berry Muffins

This is an easy and simple recipe that is low in carbs.

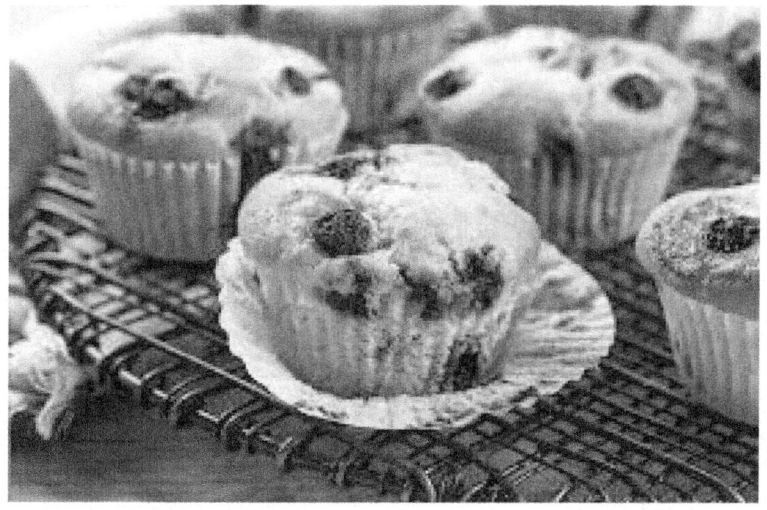

- Total Time: 40 mins

- Prep. Time: 10 mins

- Cooking Time: 30 mins

- Serving size: 4 servings

Ingredients:

1. 100 g blueberries

2. 1 cup almond flour

3. 4 tbsp butter

4. ½ cup milk

5. 2 eggs

6. 1 tsp baking powder

7. ½ cup honey

Instructions:

- In a bowl whisk eggs and add milk.

- Mix well, and then add honey and melted butter. Take care that the butter should not be warm.

- Preheat oven to 400∘F.

- Prepare a muffin tray and apply a thin layer of oil to it.

- In the egg mixture, add all the dry ingredients and add the blueberries.

- Make a smooth batter.

- Scoop the batter into the muffin tray and bake for 30 mins.

- When the muffins are baked, let them rest for 10 to 15 mins before serving.

6.8. Mango Ice Cream

This is one-ingredient ice cream. It is easy to make and is as delicious as store-bought mango ice cream.

- Total Time: 15 mins

- Prep. Time: 5 mins

- Cooking Time: N/A

- Serving Size: 3 servings

Ingredients:

1. 3 mangoes

Instructions:

- Peel and slice the mangoes and store them in a zip lock bag in a freezer for 3 hours.
- Take out from the freezer and add to a food processor and start pulsing at the highest speed.
- You will see after 3 to 4 mins the pieces will start to form chunks.
- Next, open the processor and scrape the mangoes from the corners.
- Again, start pulsing, and you will see the banana will form oatmeal consistency.
- Again, scrape the mango from the corners.
- Keep pulsing, and you will see a creamy texture starts forming.
- Blend for 2 more minutes and scoop the ice cream.
- Enjoy your 1 ingredient ice cream.

6.9. Strawberry Trifle

This is a sweet and tangy dessert. It has the right amount of sweetness which is complemented by the tangy flavor of strawberry.

- Total Time: 30 mins
- Prep. Time: 15 mins
- Cooking Time: 10 mins
- Serving Size: 4 servings

Ingredients:

1. 2oo g plain cake slices
2. 1 pack of strawberry jelly
3. 100 g fresh strawberries sliced.
4. 2 tsp sugar
5. 4 tbsp vanilla custard powder
6. 6 tbsp honey
7. 750 ml milk

Instructions:

- Slice the strawberries and put them in a saucepan. Add 2 tsp sugar and cook on light flame for 2 mins till the strawberry leaves the water. Set aside.

- In a large saucepan, pour milk and bring to boil. Take out some milk in a cup, mix the custard powder, and pour it back to the saucepan. Cook for 2 minutes and add the honey. Mix well. Keep it in the fridge to cool for 20 mins.

- Take two cups of water and bring to boil, add the jelly crystals, and mix well. Take the saucepan off the stove.

- Pour it into a glass container and keep it in the refrigerator to cool.

- Next, take a rectangle-shaped serving tray and put in the plain cake to form the bottom layer.

- On the top of the cake spread the strawberries.

- On top of that layer, pour the thick custard.

- Next, cut the jelly into cubes and spread it over the custard.

- Enjoy your strawberry trifle.

6.10. Avocado Brownies

This is an amazing recipe with low calories and doubles the flavor.

- Total Time: 40 mins
- Prep. Time: 5 mins
- Cooking Time: 35 mins
- Serving Size: 4 servings

Ingredients:

1. 1 ripe avocado
2. 2 bananas
3. ¼ cup maple syrup
4. 1 cup coconut flour
5. 3 eggs

6. ½ cup coco powder

7. 1 tsp baking powder

8. 2 tbsp chocolate chips

Instructions:

- Cut the avocado and take out the pulp with a spoon. Put it in a large mixing bowl.

- Peel the bananas and put them in the mixing bowl.

- Add all the other ingredients and mix well.

- Put everything in a blender and make a batter.

- Preheat the oven at 300 ∘F. Prepare a square baking dish with butter paper.

- Pour the batter into the baking dish and bake for 35 mins.

- When the brownies are baked, let them cool down before cutting and serving.

- You can serve with homemade banana or mango ice cream.

6.11. Pineapple Delight

- Total Time: 30 mins

- Prep. Time: 15 mins

- Cooking Time: 10 mins

- Serving Size: 4 servings

Ingredients:

1. 2oo g plain cake slices

2. 1 pack of pineapple jelly

3. 100 g canned pineapple sliced.

4. 2 tsp sugar

5. 4 tbsp vanilla custard powder

6. 6 tbsp honey

7. 750 ml milk

Instructions:

- In a large saucepan, pour milk and bring to boil. Take out some milk in a cup, mix the custard powder, and pour it back to the saucepan. Cook for 2 minutes and add the honey. Mix well. Keep it in the fridge to cool for 20 mins.

- Take two cups of water and bring to boil, add the jelly crystals, and mix well. Take the saucepan off the stove.

- Pour it into a glass container and keep it in the refrigerator to cool.

- Next, take a rectangle-shaped serving tray and put in the plain cake to form the bottom layer. Pour 3 tbsp of pineapple juice from the can on the cake.

- On the top of the cake spread the pineapple.

- On top of that layer, pour the thick custard.

- Next, cut the jelly into cubes and spread it over the custard.

- Enjoy your strawberry trifle.

6.12. Pecan Pie

- Total Time: 1 hour 15 mins

- Prep time: 15 mins

- Cook time: 50 mins.

- Serving size: 8 servings

Ingredients

1. 1 cup chopped pecans.

2. ½ cup butter

3. ¾ cup brown sugar

4. 2 eggs

5. ½ cup white sugar

6. 2 tablespoon flour

7. 2 tablespoon milk

8. 1 teaspoon vanilla extract

Instructions

- Preheat oven to 375 °F.

- Prepare a 9-inch pie dish by greasing it with oil.

- Beat eggs in a large bowl until a foamy consistency is achieved.

- Stir in the butter. After that, add white sugar, brown sugar, and flour; mix well. In the end, add vanilla, milk, and nuts.

- Pour in the pie dish.

- Bake in preheated oven for 10 minutes.

- Reduce temperature to 325 °F and then bake again for 30 to 40 minutes, or until done.

- Serve when cooled to room temperature.

6.13. Chocolate Bombs:

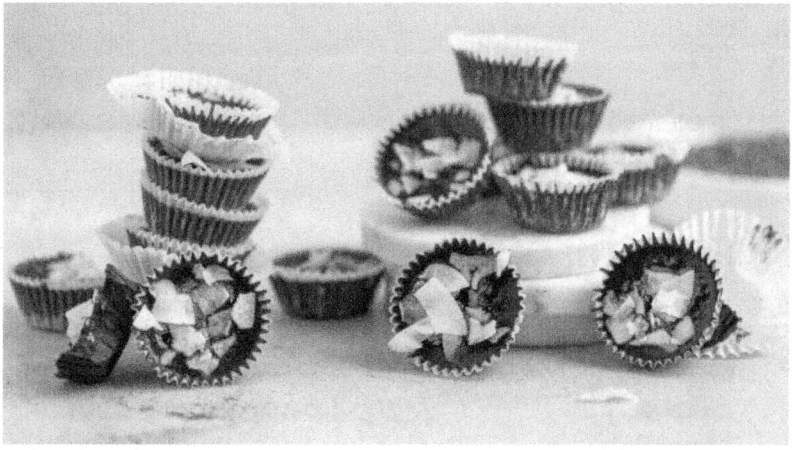

- Total Time: 30 minutes

- Prep. Time: 10 mins

- Cooking Time: 20 mins

- Serving Size: 6 servings

Ingredients:

1. ¾ cup coco powder

2. ¾ cup of coconut oil

3. ¾ cup peanut butter

4. ½ cup coconut shavings

5. 25 g brown sugar

6. ½ tsp salt

7. ½ tsp cayenne pepper

8. 1 tsp cinnamon powder

Instructions:

- Prepare a muffin tray with cupcake liners.

- Preheat the oven to 300∘F.

- Mix the coco powder, oil and peanut butter in a glass bowl, and heat over a water bath till a smooth mixture is formed.

- Mix in it the salt, cinnamon powder, sugar, and cayenne pepper.

- Mix well, and when the batter is formed, scoop it into the muffin tray.

- Bake for 20 minutes.

- Take out the chocolate bombs and top with coconut shavings.

6.14. Chocolate Chip Cookie

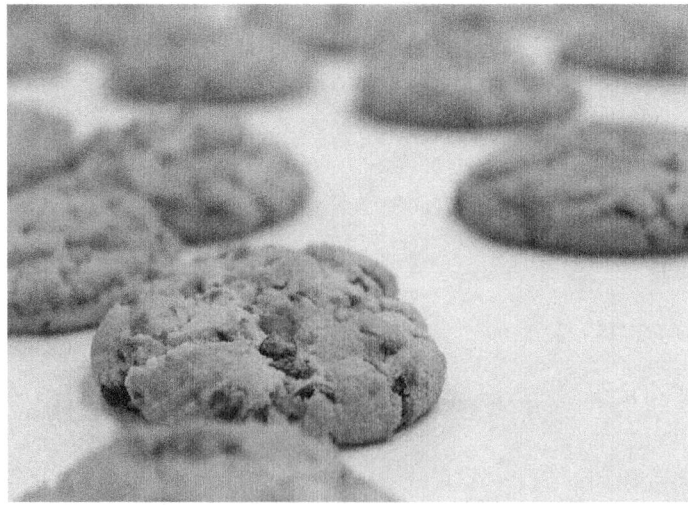

- Total Time: 1 hour 5 mins

- Prep. time: 45 mins

- Cooking time: 20 mins
- Serving size: 36 servings

Ingredients:

1. 2 ½ cup flour
2. 2 eggs
3. ½ cup ground oats
4. 1 cup brown sugar
5. ½ cup white sugar
6. ¾ cup unsalted butter
7. 200g English toffee bits
8. 200g chocolate chips
9. 1 tsp vanilla essence
10. 1 tsp baking powder
11. ½ tsp salt

Instructions:

- Preheat oven at 300 °F.
- Prepare a cookie tray by lining it with butter paper.
- Put the oats in a food processor. Grind them finely.
- Put the brown and white sugar with the vanilla essence in a large bowl and mix with an electric mixer.
- While mixing, add the melted butter to the mixture. Keep on mixing and add the eggs. Put inside the baking powder and salt. Keep mixing. Slowly add powdered oats and flour. In the end, add the chocolate chips and toffee bits.
- Now chill this dough. The method to chill will be by shaping the dough into a log and wrap in butter paper.
- After 30 minutes, cut the dough into rounds with a knife.
- Bake for 10-12 minutes or until the edges are brown and the middle looks slightly underbaked. Take out the tray from the oven and cool to room temperature.

- You can also freeze the dough for up to a month. The baking time for frozen dough is 10 minutes more than when you use the chilled dough.

6.15. Zesty Cheesecake

- Total Time: 1 hour 40 mins

- Prep time: 15 mins

- Cooking time: 1 hour 25 mins

- Serving size: 8 servings

Ingredients:

1. 2 cups graham cracker crumbs

2. 3 eggs

3. 600g cream cheese

4. 150g sour cream

5. 1/3 cup cream

6. 1 ½ tbsp lemon rind

7. 1/3 cup butter

8. 1 cup sugar

9. 1 tsp vanilla essence

Instructions:

- Preheat the oven to 225°F.

- In a bowl, mix melted butter, graham cracker crumbs, sugar and press into the removable pan.

- Bake for 10 minutes.

- Turn the oven off and remove the pan and allow it to cool completely.

- Mix the cream cheese and sugar using an electric mixer.

- Add the sour cream, lemon rind, and vanilla and mix until combined.

- Add the cream and eggs and mix until smooth.

- Pour into the springform pan.

- Cover the entire springform pan with plastic wrap, wrapping it in the container two times. The cling wrap should cover the pan fully.

- Place the pan into the oven. Set the oven to Convection Mode at 225°F.

- Bake for 1 hour and 15 minutes.

6.16. Tangy Lemon Bars

- Total Time: 5o mins

- Prep time: 15 minutes

- Cooking time: 35 minutes

- Serving size: 8 servings

Ingredients:

1. 2 ½ cup flour

2. 3 eggs

3. 2 cup sugar

4. 4 tsp lemon zest

5. 100g butter

6. ¼ cup lemon juice

Instructions:

- Preheat the oven to 325 °F.

- Prepare a rectangle pan by greasing it with oil.

- Mix all ingredients in a food processor and mix them till the ingredients look sandy a mixture.

- In a large bowl, take the sandy mixture out and knead it till a dough is formed.

- Press this dough in the baking pan and bake for 15-20 minutes.

- Take out from the oven and let it cool completely.

- Do not turn off the oven.

- Mix sugar and flour in a large bowl.

- Add all the ingredients left and mix to form a uniform mixture.

- Pour this mixture over the already baked dough.

- Bake for 12-15 minutes.

- Take out from the oven. Let it cool before serving.

6.17. Caramel Square Sweet

- Total Time: 35 mins

- Prep time: 10 mins

- Cook time: 25 mins.

- Serving size: 10 servings

Ingredients:

1. 1 ½ almond flour

2. 2 tsp baking powder

3. ½ cup brown sugar

4. 25 store brought caramel cubes.

5. 1/2 tsp baking powder

6. ½ cup butter

7. ¼ cup milk

8. 100g chocolate chips

9. Pinch of salt

Instructions:

- Preheat oven at 340°F.

- Prepare a rectangular baking tray by greasing it with oil. The size could be 13 inches by 9 inches or any size near this range.

- In a large bowl, mix brown sugar, oats, flour, baking powder, and salt. Mix the butter in sections and check the mixture. Stop adding butter when a crumbly mixture is formed.

- Set one cup of the mixture aside for later use.

- Put the remaining mixture in the baking tray and press down.

- Place the pan on the middle rack of the oven and bake for 10-12 minutes or till the mixture becomes bubbly. Take out the tray from the oven and let it cool.

- In a saucepan, mix the caramel squares and milk. Melt the mixture on low flame. When it is fully melted, add two tablespoons of flour to the mixture.

- Next, pour the caramel syrup carefully on the crust.

- Spread the chocolate chips in a single layer on the caramel layer.

- Put a layer of remaining dough on top of the chocolate chips and press evenly.

- Put the baking pan into the oven for 10-12 minutes.

- Take out the pan and let it cool.

- Cut into squares and serve.

6.18. Fudge Brownies

- Total Time: 55 mins

- Prep time: 15 mins

- Cooking time: 40 mins

- Serving size: 8 servings

Ingredients:

1. 1 ½ cups butter, melted.

2. 6 eggs

3. 2 cup flour

4. 3 cup sugar

5. 1 tbsp vanilla essence

6. 1 ¼ cup cocoa powder

7. 1 tbsp salt

Instructions:

- Preheat the oven to 325 °F.

- We will be using the center position rack for baking in this recipe.

- Grease a rectangle baking pan for this recipe. The size can be 13 inches by 9 inches or somewhere near this size.

- Mix sugar, vanilla, salt, and melted butter in a large bowl and whisk till a smooth mixture is formed.

- Add the eggs to this mixture.

- Sift coco powder and flour in a bowl.

- Fold the flour and coco powder into this mixture. Make a smooth batter.

- Pour this into the already prepared baking pan.

- Bake for 35-40 minutes. Check for doneness.

- It can be served warm with vanilla ice cream.

6.19. Jam Cookies

- Total Time: 25 mins

- Prep time: 10 mins

- Cook time: 15 mins.

- Serving size: 12 servings

Ingredients:

1. 1 ½ cup softened butter.

2. 2 ½ cup flour

3. 3 egg yolks

4. 1 cup sugar

5. 1 tsp vanilla

6. 1 1/2 tsp salt

7. 1 jar strawberry jam

Instructions:

- First, preheat the oven to 325 °F.

- Line a cookie tray with butter paper.

- In a large mixing bowl, put butter, salt, sugar, and vanilla. Use an electric beater or stand mixer to make a smooth mixture.

- To this mixture, add the egg yolks and mix for 2 minutes till the egg yolk is fully incorporated.

- Fold in the flour to the mixture with a wooden spoon. Mix till the flour is incorporated.

- With a 1-inch scoop, make 12 balls of the dough and place it on the baking tray.

- Wet your hands and make a depression in each ball with the thumb.

- With a spoon, put a small quantity of jam into each thumb depression.

- Bake the cookies for 10-12 minutes.

- Repeat the entire process with the dough that is left. You can prepare multiple trays and bake them simultaneously on different racks of the oven.

6.20. Apple pie

- Total Time: 40 mins

- Prep time: 20 mins

- Cook time: 20 mins.

- Serving size: 6 servings

Ingredients:

1. 125g brown sugar

2. 2 tbsp white sugar

3. ¼ cup almond flour

4. Store-bought pastry dough

5. 1 kg apples

6. 5 strips of orange zest (1 inch thick)

7. 1 cup water

8. ½ tsp cinnamon

9. ¼ tsp allspice

10. 2 tbsp milk

Instructions:

- First, preheat the oven to 400 °F.

- Put a large and heavy baking tray in the middle rack of the oven.

- In a saucepan, put the brown sugar salt, water, zest, cinnamon, and allspice and put it on the stove on high till all the sugar is dissolved in water completely.

- Lower flame and cook till a thick syrup are formed. It should be almost reduced to ¾ cup. Remove the zest with a spoon or pass through a sieve. Let the syrup cool for 2 to 3 minutes.

- Peel apples, remove the seeds and cut them into half-inch wedges.

- Take a bowl and pour flour into it. Coat the apples with flour and dip them in the syrup. Set the apple slices in a separate bowl.

- Roll out the dough for a nine-inch pie dish. Put in the pie dish, and chill.

- Roll out another piece of dough in a 15- inch by 10- inch rectangle. Cut dough into strips lengthwise.

- Put the apples on the pie crust.

- Trim the strips to the size of the pie dish. Make a lattice on the top of the pie with the stripes.

- Wash the lattice by brushing some egg while and then some milk.

- Place the pie dish on the already preheated baking tray.

- Bake for 20 minutes.

- Check for doneness. It is done when the crusts are light brown.

- Serve warm.

6.21. Cookie Bars

- Total Time: 35 mins
- Prep time: 10 mins
- Cooking time: 25 mins
- Serving size: 25 servings

Ingredients:

1. 6 tbsp salted butter
2. 1 cup chopped cherries.
3. 1 cup flaked unsweetened coconut.
4. 1 ½ cup of cooking chocolate crumbs
5. 1liter condensed milk (sweetened)
6. 1 cup of chocolate chips

Instructions:

- Preheat your oven to 325° F.
- Prepare a square pan,8x8 inches. Line the pan first with aluminum foil for easy removal of material after baking.
- Spread all the butter on the base of the baking pan.
- Put the chocolate crumbs on top of the butter in a single layer.
- Pour the condensed milk on the crumbs and form an even layer.
- Make a layer of cherries on top of condensed milk.
- Then make a layer of coconut over it. All layers should be even.
- In the end, make a layer of chocolate chips. Press gently.
- Bake in the oven for 20-25 minutes or until the coconut changes to a golden brown.
- Remove from the oven.
- Let it cool completely in the baking pan.
- After it has reached room temperature, slice to bars.

- It can be served at room temperature or after refrigeration.

6.22. Almond Cookies

- Total Time: 30 mins
- Prep time: 15 mins
- Cook time: 15 mins.
- Serving size: 32 pieces

Ingredients:

1. 226.8 g unsalted butter
2. 112 g almond flour
3. 2 cups flour
4. 2 tsp vanilla essence
5. 1 ½ cups icing sugar.
6. 1 tsp orange zest

Instructions:

- First, preheat the oven to 350 °F.
- Line a large cookie tray with butter paper.
- In a large bowl, beat the sugar, vanilla essence, and butter. Use an electric beater or stand mixer. Form a smooth mixture.
- Now with a wooden spoon, fold in the flour and salt. When this is mixed properly, add the almond flour, and fold it in the same way. Take care that no lumps are formed. Add the orange zest and mix well. If the batter is sticky, add a bit of flour but not too much, just enough so that dough is formed and is not sticky anymore.
- Form the dough into small balls. You can use a small 1-inch scoop to make the balls.
- Put them on a prepared baking tray. The balls should be 1-inch apart.
- You should get 35-40 cookies. Do not make them too large or too small. Large balls will not bake properly, and small balls will become hard.

- Bake for 10-12 minutes. Take out from the oven and let it cool just for 5 minutes.

- Put the icing sugar in a medium-size bowl and roll the cookies in the sugar. This should be done when the balls are still a bit warm.

- Transfer all the cookies to a separate tray and let them cool to room temperature.

- Roll the cookies again in the icing sugar to give a snowball-like look.

6.23. Coco Marble Cake

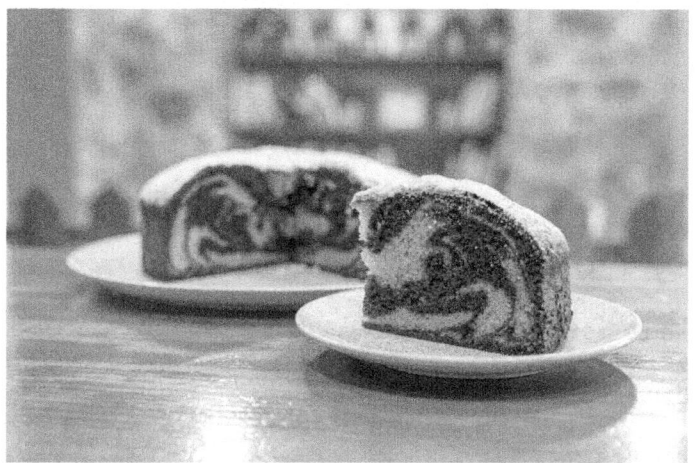

- Total Time: 40 mins

- Prep time: 10 mins

- Cook time: 30 mins.

- Serving size: 5 servings

Ingredients:

1. 3 eggs

2. 1 cup flour

3. 1 tsp baking powder

4. ¾ cup vegetable oil

5. 1 cup sugar

6. 2 tbsp coco powder

7. 1 tsp vanilla essence

Instructions:

- Preheat oven at 300 °F.

- Prepare a round cake tin by greasing it with oil.

- In a mixing bowl, separate three egg whites. Set the yolks aside. Beat the egg whites so much that a cloud consistency is attained.

- Mix the yolks and oil into the mixture.

- Then add sugar and mix well.

- Lastly, fold the flour in parts to the mixture so that lumps are not formed.

- When a smooth mixture is achieved, in a small cup, separate four tablespoons of mixture.

- Pour the batter from the mixing bowl into the baking tin.

- To the batter in the cup, add the coco powder and mix well

- Add this coco mixture to the baking tin and give it a swirl with the spoon.

- Bake for 30 minutes.

- Dust with icing sugar

- Serve after refrigeration.

6.24. Raisin Cookies

- Total Time: 30 mins

- Prep time: 20 mins

- Cooking time: 10 mins

- Serving size: 48 servings

Ingredients:

1. 1 ½ cup flour

2. 3 cups rolled oats.

3. 1 cup black raisins

4. 1 cup butter

5. 2 eggs

6. 220g white sugar

7. 220 g brown sugar

8. 1 tablespoon vanilla essence

9. ½ teaspoon baking powder

10. 1 teaspoon ground cinnamon

11. 1 teaspoon salt

Instructions:

- First, preheat the oven to 350 °F.

- Prepare a large cookie sheet with butter paper.

- In a large bowl, use an electric beater to mix the white sugar, butter, and brown sugar until a silky and smooth mixture is formed. Add in the vanilla essence and eggs until a fluffy consistency is achieved.

- In a separate bowl, mix baking powder, cinnamon, flour, and salt. Slowly beat into the egg batter.

- Add in the oats and raisins by hand. The dough should be formed.

- Put tablespoonfuls of the dough on the cookie tray at a 2-inch distance. This will ensure space for the cookie to expand while baking. Each cookie will remain separate. If we dump the cookie dough near, they will all become joined after baking.

- Bake for 10-12 minutes.

- Check for doneness. The cookies should be golden brown.

- Let the cookies cool before use. These can be stored for up to a month.

6.25. Pistachio Biscotti

- Total Time: 1 hour 15 mins

- Prep time: 25 mins

- Cook time:45 mins.

- Serving size: 36 servings

Ingredients:

1. 1 cup pistachio nuts
2. ½ cup dried cranberries
3. 2 cups flour
4. 2 eggs
5. 2 tablespoon olive oil
6. ¾ cup white sugar
7. 1 teaspoon baking powder
8. 2 teaspoons vanilla essence
9. 1 teaspoon almond essence
10. ¼ teaspoon salt

Instructions:

- Preheat the oven to 300 °F.
- Prepare a large cookie tray by lining it with butter paper.
- Combine the sugar and oil in a large bowl. Use a blender to mix till a uniform mixture is formed.
- Add to the mixture almond essence, vanilla essence, and eggs.
- In a separate bowl, make the baking powder, flour, and salt. Slowly fold this powder mix into the egg batter. No lumps should be formed.
- Add the cranberries and nuts on top and give a light stir to mix.
- Divide this batter into two. Shape two logs on the prepared cookie tray. They should be approximately 10x3 inches each.
- The dough can be a little be loose. So, wet hands with cold water to form the logs easily.
- Bake for 30 minutes in the preheated oven.
- Check the logs for doneness. They should be light brown on the outside.

- Take them out from the oven and leave to cool for 10 minutes.

- Next, lower the temperature of the oven to 250°F.

- Cut the cookie logs into 1-inch-thick slices.

- Remove the old butter paper from the cookie tray and line it with new.

- Lay the 1-inch pieces on the cookie tray.

- Bake for 10-12 minutes.

- Check for doneness. The biscotti should be dry but still easily breakable.

- Let it cool.

- Use immediately or keep for later. It can be used for up to a month.

6.26. Orange Cake

- Total Time: 1 hour 30 mins

- Prep time: 30 mins

- Cooking time: 1 hour

- Serving size: 8 servings

Ingredients:

1. 250g packet yellow cake mix.

2. 50g package instant lemon pudding mix

3. 4 eggs

4. 2 tablespoon butter

5. 1 cup orange juice

6. ½ cup vegetable oil

7. 1 teaspoon lemon essence

8. ⅔ cup white sugar

Instructions:

- Preheat oven to 300 °F.

- Prepare a 10-inch Bundt baking pan by oiling it.

- In a large bowl, mix the pudding mix and cake.

- Make a space in the middle of the powder mix and add 1 cup orange juice, eggs, lemon essence, and oil. Beat in low speed with a hand blender or a stand blender.

- Using a spatula, takes the material off from the bowl sizes and blends again until a uniform mixture is formed.

- Put the mixture in the already prepared baking pan.

- Bake for 50-60 minutes.

- Check for doneness and take out of the oven.

- Let the cake cool.

- Meanwhile, make the orange sauce.

- In a pan, add six tablespoons of orange juice, butter, and sugar. Heat it on a medium flame for 1 minute. Pour this mixture over the cake.

- Serve either warm or chilled.

6.27. Chocolate Chip Cake

- Total Time: 40 mins

- Prep time: 10 mins

- Cooking time: 30 mins

- Serving size: 6 servings

Ingredients:

1. 3 eggs

2. 1 cup flour

3. 1 tsp baking powder

4. ¾ cup vegetable oil

5. 1 cup sugar

6. 4 tbsp coco powder

7. 1 tbsp vanilla essence

8. ½ cup chocolate chips

Instructions:

- Preheat oven at 300 °F.

- Prepare a round cake tin by greasing it with oil.

- In a mixing bowl, separate 3 egg whites. Set the yolks aside. Beat the egg whites so much that a cloud consistency is attained.

- Mix the yolks and oil into the mixture.

- Then add sugar and mix well.

- Lastly, fold the flour in parts to the mixture so that lumps are not formed. Fold in the coco powder and form a silky and smooth batter.

- Pour the batter from the mixing bowl into the baking tin.

- Sprinkle the chocolate chips on the batter.

- Bake for 30 minutes.

- Check for doneness. After taking it out of the oven, let it cool to room temperature.

- Serve at room temperature or after refrigeration.

Chapter 7.

Drinks

Keeping hydrated is an essential part of a diet, and fasting becomes more important. In this chapter, there are recipes for easy and simple drinks that can be taken during the eating window of intermittent fasting.

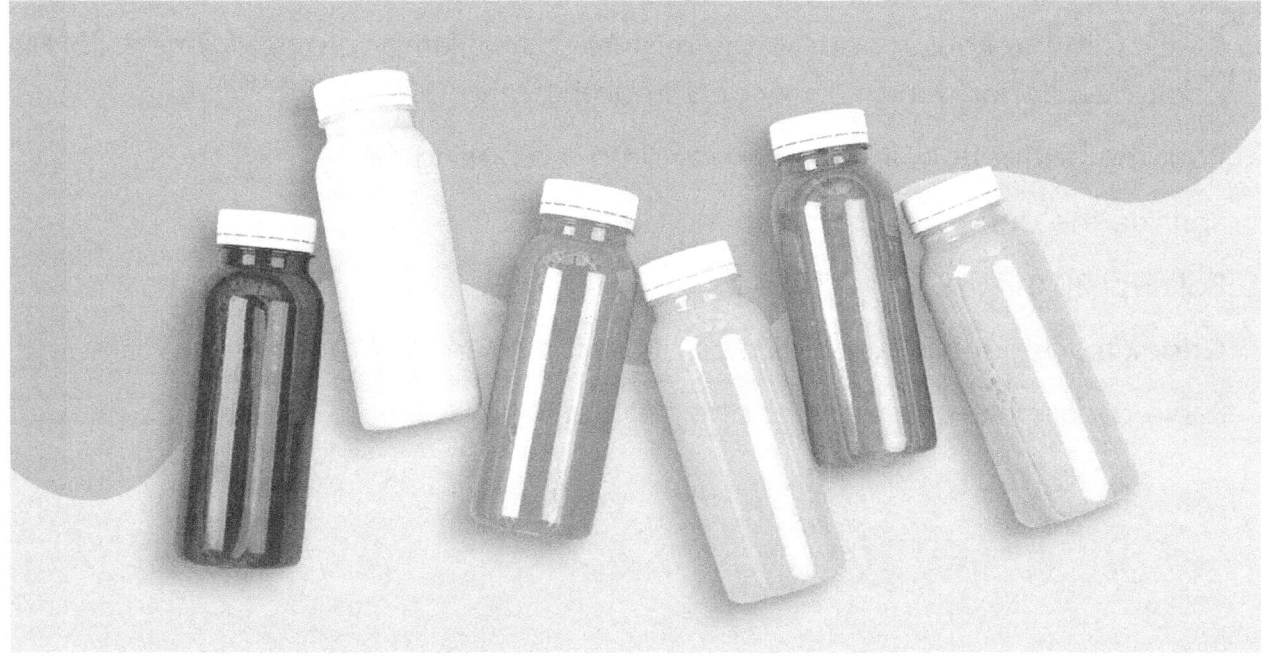

7.1. Carrot, Apple, and Orange Juice

This is a refreshing juice. It is full of antioxidants and full of flavor.

- Total Time: 15 mins
- Prep. Time: 15 mins
- Cooking Time: N/A
- Serving Size: 1 serving

Ingredients:

1. 2 apples
2. 2 carrots
3. 2 oranges
4. 1 pinch salt
5. 1 pinch pepper

Instructions:

- Cut the apples and carrots. Remove the apple seeds. Juice the apples and carrots with a juicer machine. Collect the juice in a glass.

- Cut the oranges in half. Squeeze the orange juice into the orange and apple juice mix. Or use a machine to juice the oranges and mix them into the other fruit juices.

- Add a pinch of salt and pepper to the juice to enhance the taste.

- Enjoy your juice.

7.2. Strawberry Smoothie

Strawberries are refreshing and provide essential vitamins. Yogurt is a good source of calcium. This recipe is perfect for consuming bone and gut health.

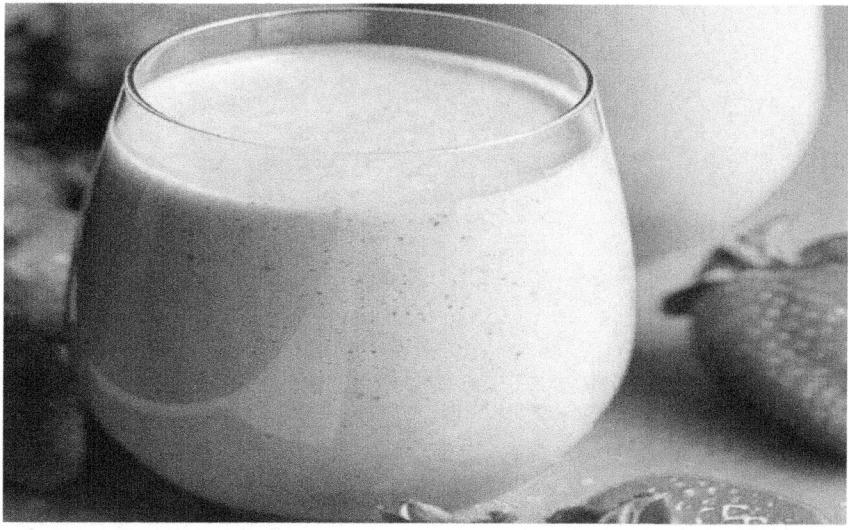

- Total Time: 5 mins

- Prep. Time: 5 mins

- Cooking Time: N/A
- Serving Size: 1 serving

Ingredients:

1. 6 strawberries (ripe)
2. ½ cup yogurt
3. ¼ cup water
4. 1 tsp honey

Instructions:

- Put all the ingredients in a blender.
- Blend till a smooth mixture is formed.
- Add ice cubes and blend if you prefer a chilled smoothie.

7.3. Hot chocolate

Chocolate is good for weight loss if consumed in moderation, and milk is a good calcium source. This is an excellent drink for intermittent fasting, but you must keep the sugar content in check, so we use a sugar substitute.

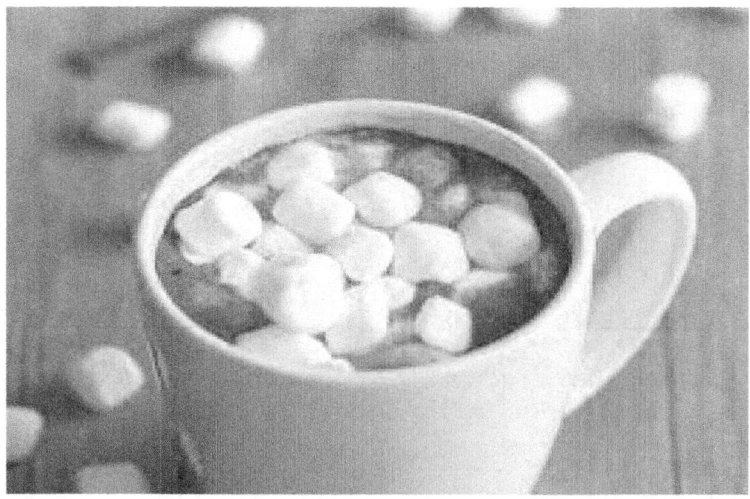

- Total Time: 5-8 mins
- Prep. Time: 3 mins
- Cooking Time: 3-4 mins

- Serving Size: 1 serving

Ingredients:

1. 1 cup milk

2. 1 tsp coco powder

3. 1 tsp Splenda sugar

4. 2 tsp mini marshmallows

Instructions:

- In a small saucepan, bring milk to boil and add the coco powder. Let it mix and cook for 2 minutes.

- Pour the hot chocolate into a cup, add Splenda sugar and top with marshmallows.

- This drink is much enjoyed in the winters.

7.4. Coffee

For some people, coffee is essential to kick-start their day. You cannot consume anything except the black coffee version during the fast, but you can have a warm cup of milk coffee during your eating window.

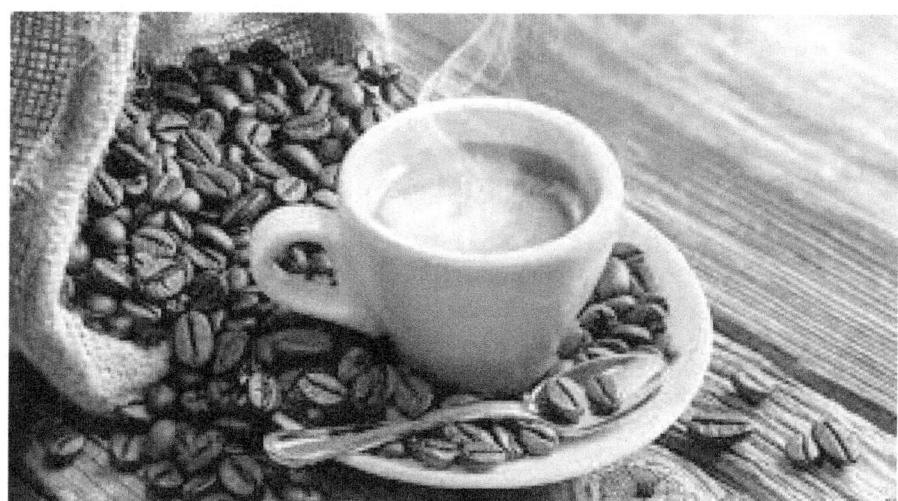

- Total Time: 10 mins

- Prep. Time: 5 mins

- Cooking Time: 5 mins

- Serving Size: 1 serving

Ingredients:

1. 1 tsp ground coffee
2. 1 cup milk
3. 1 tsp sugar
4. 3 tsp water

Instructions:

- In a mug, add the coffee, sugar, and water and a spoon mix.
- Keep mixing till a smooth mixture is formed, and the coffee and sugar are fully dissolved.
- Now boil one cup of milk and pour it over the coffee.
- Mix well. Enjoy your cup of coffee.

7.5. Chamomile Latte

This latte is a caffeine-free beverage if your target is also to cut down on your caffeine intake. This can be a good option to break your fast.

- Total Time: 20 mins
- Prep Time: 2 mins
- Cooking Time: 5 mins
- Serving size: 1 serving

Ingredients:

1. 1 tsp dried chamomile flower n leaves
2. 1 ½ cup almond milk
3. 1 tsp honey
4. ¼ tsp cinnamon
5. 1 pinch clove powder

Instructions:

- In a saucepan, add the almond milk and chamomile and bring to boil. Let it boil for 2 minutes. Then, turn off the stove and cover the saucepan. Let the tea infuse for 5-10 mins.

- After 10 mins, strain the tea in a cup and top it with cinnamon and clove powder. Add honey for sweetness.

7.6. Chocolate Strawberry Shake

This is a cold chocolate shake that has a creamy texture and delicious flavor.

- Total Time: 5 mins

- Prep Time: 5 mins

- Cooking Time: N/A

- Serving Size: 1 serving

Ingredients:

1. 1 tsp coco powder

2. 3 strawberries

3. ½ cup milk

4. ½ cup yogurt

5. 2 tsp honey

Instructions:

- Add all the ingredients to a blender.

- Blend till a homogeneous shake is formed.

- Add ice cubes and blend for 2 to 3 minutes for a chilling effect.

7.7. Banana Smoothie

Banana is one of the most popular foods in the world. Banana is a whole meal and a good source of vitamin K.

- Total Time: 10 mins

- Prep Time: 5 mins
- Cooking Time: N/A
- Serving Size: 1 serving

Ingredients:

1. 1 ripe banana
2. ½ cup Greek yogurt
3. ¼ cup milk
4. 1 tsp chia seeds
5. 1 tsp flax seeds

Instructions:

- Add all the ingredients to a blender.
- Blend till a thick smoothie is formed.
- Add ice cubes and blend for 3 minutes for a chilling effect.

7.8. Watermelon Chill

Watermelon is a refreshing fruit and hydrates the body and skin. This is a simple recipe to make a chilled watermelon drink.

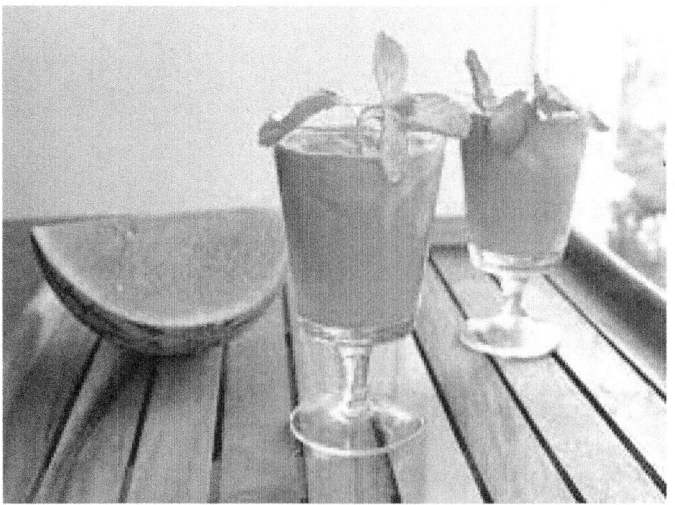

- Total Time: 10 mins
- Prep Time: 5 mins

- Cooking Time: N/A
- Serving Size: 2 servings

Ingredients:

1. ½ small watermelon
2. Few mint leaves
3. ¼ tsp salt
4. ¼ tsp pepper
5. 2 tbsp lemon juice

Instructions:

- Take out the pulp of half of the watermelon and remove the seeds.
- Cut into small pieces and put them in a blender. Add the mint leaves, salt, pepper, and lemon juice.
- Blend well.
- Add ice cubes to the blender and blend for 3 to 4 mins.
- Serve cold.

7.9. Pina Colada

This is a famous drink for summer days. Here is a simple recipe for a pina colada.

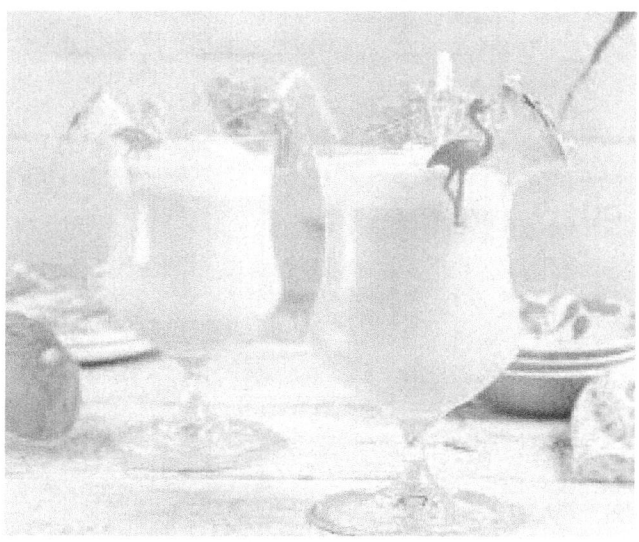

- Total Time: 10 mins
- Prep. Time: 5 mins
- Cooking Time: N/A
- Serving Size: 2 servings

Ingredients:

1. 1 ½ cup pineapple juice
2. ¾ cup coconut milk
3. 1 tsp grated coconut
4. Few pineapple pieces for decoration

Instructions:

- In a jug, mix the pineapple juice and coconut milk. Mix well and add the grated coconut.
- Put it in the blender and add ice cubes. Blend for 2 mins.
- Pour in glasses and decorate with pineapples on the glass edges.

7.10. Peach Smoothie

When you are following intermittent fasting, you should include fresh fruits in your diet. This recipe incorporates fresh fruit and yogurt, which is a great source of calcium.

- Total Time: 5 mins
- Prep. Time: 5 mins
- Cooking Time: N/A
- Serving Size: 1 serving

Ingredients:

1. 1 peach
2. ½ cup yogurt
3. ½ tsp honey

4. ¼ cup milk

Instructions:

- Peel the peach and cut it into pieces.

- Add the pieces to the blender with all other ingredients.

- Blend till a smoothie consistency is formed. If it is too thick, add a little more milk or water.

- All the ingredients used must be chilled for the best results.

7.11. Milk Tea

Milk tea is helpful as a source of calcium. Everyone who practices intermittent fasting should add some form of calcium to their daily diet.

- Total Time: 10 mins

- Prep. Time: 5 mins

- Cooking Time: 5 mins

- Serving Size: 2 servings

Ingredients:

1. 2 cups milk

2. ½ cup water

3. 1 tsp loose tea

4. 2 tsp honey

Instructions:

- In a saucepan, add milk and water and bring to boil.

- Add the loose tea and let it boil for 3 to 5 mins.

- Add honey and mix for 1 minute.

- Strain the tea in cups and enjoy your tea.

7.12. Mango Smoothie

Mango is a sweet and delicious fruit and can be enjoyed in any form. In this recipe, you will find an easy-to-make mango smoothie.

- Total Time: 5 mins

- Prep. Time: 5 mins

- Cooking Time: N/A

- Serving Size: 2 servings

Ingredients:

1. 1 frozen mango

2. 1 cup yogurt

3. ½ cup milk

Instructions:

- Peel the frozen mango and cut the pulp into cubes.

- Put the cubes in the blender along with yogurt and milk.

- Blend in the blender for 3 to 4 minutes till a smooth drink is formed.

- Drink while cold.

7.13. Ice Lemon Tea

This is a refreshing drink and gives you an energized feeling on a sunny summer day.

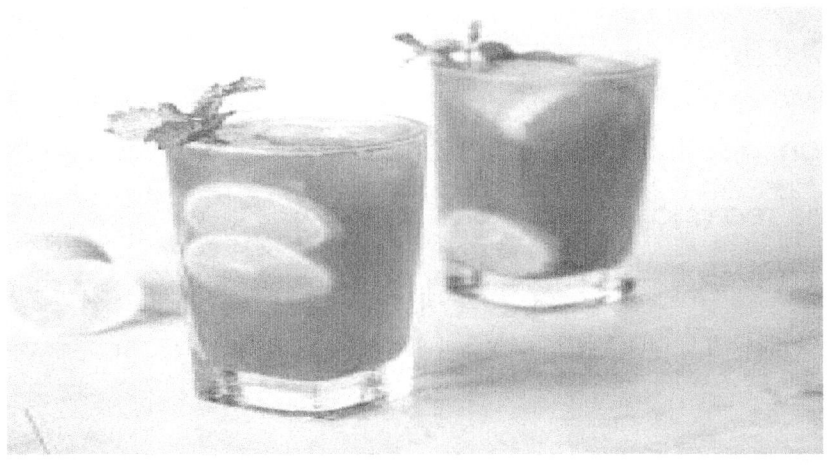

- Total Time: 15 mins

- Prep. Time: 5 mins

- Cooking Time: 5 mins

- Serving Size: 2 servings

Ingredients:

1. ½ tsp loose tea

2. 4 cups water

3. 1 sliced lemon

4. ¼ cup sugar syrup

5. 4 mint leaves for garnish

Instructions:

- Pour half a cup of water into a saucepan and bring it to boil. Add the loose tea and cook for 30 seconds.

- Please turn off the flame, strain the tea and let it cool.

- When the tea is cool, in a jug, add chilled water. To this, add tea, lemon slices and sugar syrup.

- Top with mint leaves.

- Enjoy your fresh drink.

7.14. Banana Peach Drink

This is a fruit drink that is refreshing and full of antioxidants.

- Total Time: 15 mins

- Prep. Time: 10 mins

- Cooking Time: N/A

- Serving Size: 1 serving

Ingredients:

1. 1 banana
2. 2 peaches
3. ¾ cup coconut milk
4. 1 cup chilled water.

Instructions:

- Freeze the banana and the peach in the freezer for 3 hours.
- Take out the fruits after 3 hours. Peel the fruits and slice them.
- Put the slices in the blender and add coconut milk and water.
- Blend for 5 minutes.
- Pour the juice into glasses.

7.15. Salted Lassi

Lassi is a high calcium drink that is consumed in most parts of South Asia.

- Total Time: 10 mins
- Prep. Time: 5 mins
- Cooking Time: N/A
- Serving Size: 2 serving

Ingredients:

1. 1 cup yogurt
2. 1 cup water
3. ½ tsp salt

Instructions:

- Put all the ingredients in the blender and turn on the blender.
- Blend the lassi till foam is formed on the top of the mixture.
- When the foam is formed, pour into glasses, and serve.

7.16. Sweet Lassi

- Total Time: 10 mins
- Prep. Time: 5 mins
- Cooking Time: N/A
- Serving Size: 2 serving

Ingredients:

1. 1 cup yogurt
2. 1 cup water
3. 2 tsp sugar

Instructions:

- Put all the ingredients in the blender and turn on the blender.
- Blend the lassi till foam is formed on the top of the mixture.
- When the foam is formed, pour into glasses, and serve.

7.17. Mango Lassi

- Total Time: 10 mins
- Prep. Time: 5 mins
- Cooking Time: N/A
- Serving Size: 2 serving

Ingredients:

1. 1 cup yogurt
2. 1 cup water
3. 2 tsp sugar
4. 1 mango peeled and cut into cubes.

Instructions:

- Put all the ingredients in the blender and turn on the blender.

- Blend the lassi till foam is formed on the top of the mixture.

- When the foam is formed, pour into glasses, and serve.

7.18. Banana Milkshake

- Total Time: 10 mins

- Prep Time: 5 mins

- Cooking Time: N/A

- Serving Size: 1 serving

Ingredients:

1. 1 ripe banana

2. 1 ½ cup milk

3. 1 tsp chia seeds

4. 1 tsp flax seeds

Instructions:

- Add all the ingredients to a blender.

- Blend till a smooth shake is formed.

- Add ice cubes and blend for 3 minutes for a chilling effect.

7.19. Mango Milkshake

- Total Time: 10 mins

- Prep Time: 5 mins

- Cooking Time: N/A

- Serving Size: 1 serving

Ingredients:

1. 1 mango pulp

2. 1 ½ cup milk

3. 1 tsp chia seeds

4. 1 tsp flax seeds

Instructions:

- Add all the ingredients to a blender.

- Blend till a thick shake is formed.

- Add ice cubes and blend for 3 minutes for a chilling effect.

7.20. Mocha Chocolate

- Total Time: 5-8 mins

- Prep. Time: 3 mins

- Cooking Time: 3-4 mins

- Serving Size: 1 serving

Ingredients:

1. 1 cup milk

2. 1 tsp coco powder

3. 1 tsp Splenda sugar

4. 1 tsp coffee

Instructions:

- In a small saucepan, bring milk to boil and add the coco powder and coffee. Let it mix and cook for 2 minutes.

- Pour the hot chocolate into a cup, add Splenda sugar.

- This drink is much enjoyed in the winters.

7.21. Strawberry Milkshake

- Total Time: 10 mins

- Prep Time: 5 mins

- Cooking Time: N/A
- Serving Size: 1 serving

Ingredients:

1. 6 strawberries
2. 2 tsp honey
3. 1 ½ cup milk
4. 1 tsp chia seeds
5. 1 tsp flax seeds

Instructions:

- Add all the ingredients to a blender.
- Blend till a smooth shake is formed.
- Add ice cubes and blend for 3 minutes for a chilling effect.

7.22. Chilled Chocolate Shake

- Total Time: 10 mins
- Prep Time: 5 mins
- Cooking Time: N/A
- Serving Size: 1 serving

Ingredients:

1. 1 tsp cocoa powder
2. 2 tsp honey
3. 1 ½ cup milk

Instructions:

- Add all the ingredients to a blender.
- Blend till a smooth shake is formed.
- Add ice cubes and blend for 3 minutes for a chilling effect.

7.23. Salted Mint Smoothie

- Total Time: 5 mins
- Prep. Time: 5 mins
- Cooking Time: N/A
- Serving Size: 1 serving

Ingredients:

1. ½ bunch mint leaves
2. ½ cup yogurt
3. 1 tsp salt
4. ¼ cup milk

Instructions:

- Add mint leaves in the blender with all other ingredients.
- Blend till a smoothie consistency is formed. If it is too thick, add a little more milk or water.
- All the ingredients used must be chilled for the best results.

7.24. Pomegranate and Lime Juice

- Total time: 20 mins
- Prep Time: 5 mins
- Cooking Time: N/A
- Serving Size: 1 serving

Ingredients:

1. 1 ripe pomegranate
2. ¼ cup lime juice

Instructions:

- Cut the pomegranate in half and take out all the seeds.

- Juice the seeds in a juicer machine and put them in a blender.

- Add some ice cubes and lime juice.

- Blend it in a blender for 3 minutes to get a chilled drink.

7.25. Chocolate Ice-cream Shake

- Total Time: 10 mins

- Prep. Time: 10 mins

- Cooking Time: N/A

- Serving Size: 1 serving

Ingredients:

1. 1 cup milk

2. ½ cup water

3. 2 tsp sugar

4. 1 tsp protein powder

5. 1 tsp coco powder

6. 1 scoop chocolate ice cream

Instructions:

- In a blender, add water, milk, sugar, and coco powder. Blend to make a smooth mixture.

- Add protein powder and blend well.

- Add few ice cubes and blend for 2 minutes.

- Take put the shake in a glass and top it with a scoop of ice cream.

7.26. Vanilla Shake

- Total Time: 10 mins
- Prep. Time: 10 mins
- Cooking Time: N/A
- Serving Size: 1 serving

Ingredients:

1. 1 cup milk
2. ½ cup water
3. 2 tsp sugar
4. 1 tsp protein powder
5. 1 tsp vanilla extract or seeds from 1 vanilla pod
6. 1 scoop vanilla ice cream

Instructions:

- In a blender, add water, milk, sugar, and vanilla extract. Blend to make a smooth mixture.
- Add protein powder and blend well.
- Add few ice cubes and blend for 2 minutes.
- Take put the shake in a glass and top it with a scoop of ice cream.

7.27. Banana, Peach and Mango Smoothie

- Total Time: 10 mins
- Prep. Time: 10 mins
- Cooking Time: N/A
- Serving Size: 3 serving

Ingredients:

1. 1 frozen mango

2. 2 frozen bananas

3. 2 frozen peaches

4. 1 cup yogurt

5. 1 cup milk

6. 2 tsp honey

Instructions:

- Peel all the fruits and cut them into cubes.
- Put all fruit pieces in a blender and add milk, water, yogurt, and honey.

Chapter 8.

Drinks Allowed During the Fast

In intermittent fasting, you are not allowed any food or drinks that have caloric values. But you can consume water and drinks that have no caloric value. This includes water, sugar-free coffee, tea, herbal teas, and detox water. This chapter will discuss a few easy drink recipes that you can consume during the fast.

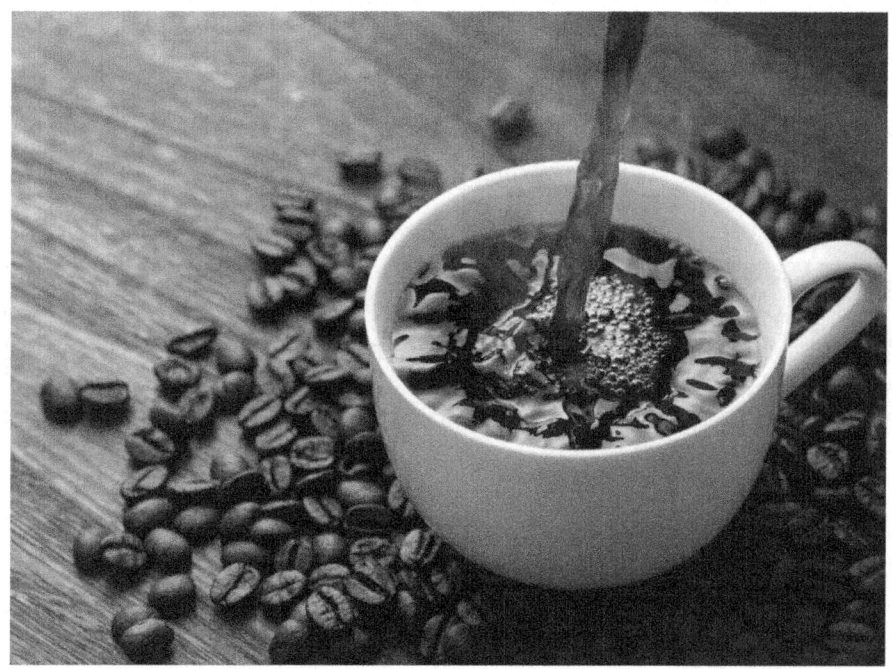

8.1. Black Coffee

This is one beverage you can consume during the fast. Usually, people who follow the 16:8 fast start their day with a cup of unsweetened black coffee.

- Total Time: 3-5 mins

- Prep. Time: N/A

- Cooking Time: 3-5 mins

- Serving Size: 1 serving

Ingredients:

1. 1 -2 tsp coffee granules
2. 1 ½ cup water

Instructions:

- In a saucepan, bring water to boil.
- Add the coffee and let the water boil for one more minute.
- Pour the coffee into your cup and enjoy.

8.2. Lemon Water

Water can be consumed during the fast as much as possible. But sometimes, a person craved for some flavor. For such a situation, lemon water is the best choice. Two ways can prepare it.

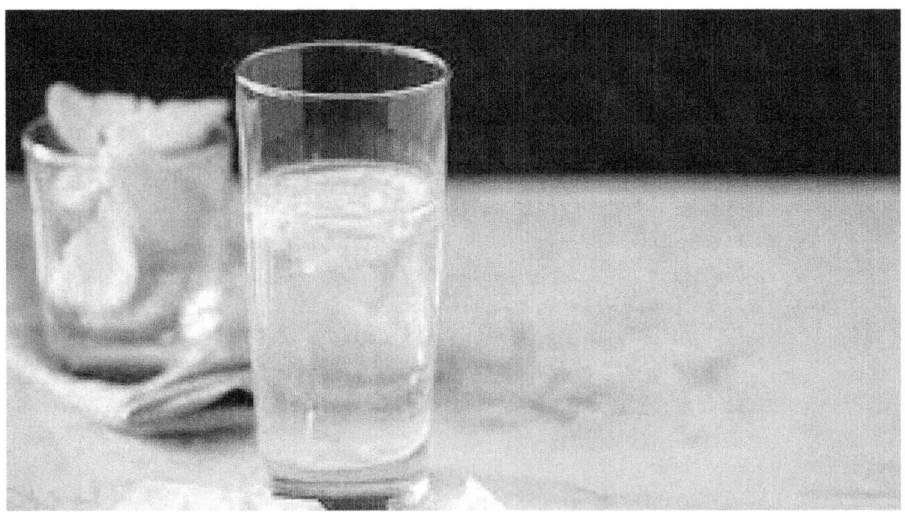

- Total Time: 5 mins
- Prep. Time: 3 mins
- Cooking Time: N/A
- Serving Size: 1 serving

Ingredients:

1. 1 lemon sliced.

2. 1 cup warm water

3. 2 tsp lemon juice

Instructions:

- In a glass or bottle, put in the lemon slices, pour the warm water over the lemons.

- Add the lemon juice and enjoy your lemon water.

- This drink also improves the metabolic rate and helps in fat burn.

8.3. Mint Tea

This tea is good for stomach health, improves metabolism, and the mint aroma has a calming effect on the body.

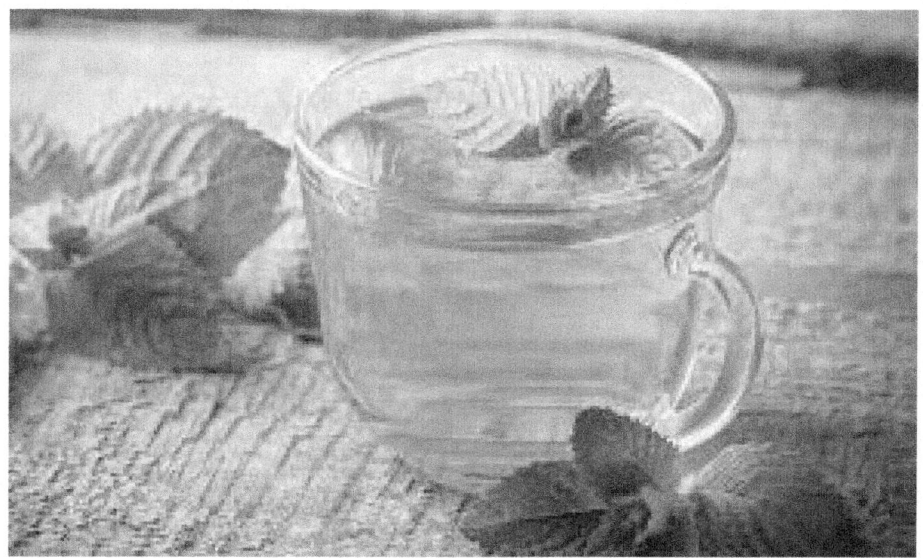

- Total Time: 5 mins

- Prep. Time: 2 mins

- Cooking Time: 3 to 4 mins

- Serving Size: 2 servings

Ingredients:

1. 5 -6 fresh mint leaves
2. ½ tsp fennel seeds
3. ½ tsp lemon juice
4. ½ tsp dry green tea or green teabag
5. 2 ½ cup water

Instructions:

- In a saucepan, bring water to boil. Add the mint leaves and fennel seeds. Let them boil for 2 minutes. Add the green tea and let it boil for ½ a minute.

- Turn off the stove and pour tea into cups.

- Add lemon juice to both cups for flavor enhancement.

8.4. Cardamom Tea

There is a bit of debate on whether tea can be consumed with milk during the fast or consumed without milk. In this recipe, we add 2 tbsp milk. It is up to you if you want to add milk or not.

- Total Time: 5-8 mins
- Prep. Time: 2 mins
- Cooking Time: 5-8 mins
- Serving Size: 2 servings

Ingredients:

1. 1 teaspoon regular breakfast tea
2. 3 cardamoms
3. 4 tbsp milk
4. 2 ½ cup water

Instructions:

- Bring water to boil and add the tea. Let the color appear.

- Break the cardamoms and add to the boiling tea. Let the tea boil for 2 minutes.

- Add the milk and again bring to boil.

- Strain the tea and pour it into the cup.

- Serve hot.

- You can skip the milk if you want.

8.5. Cucumber Water

This is great detox water. Gives you freshness and gets rid of toxins in your skin.

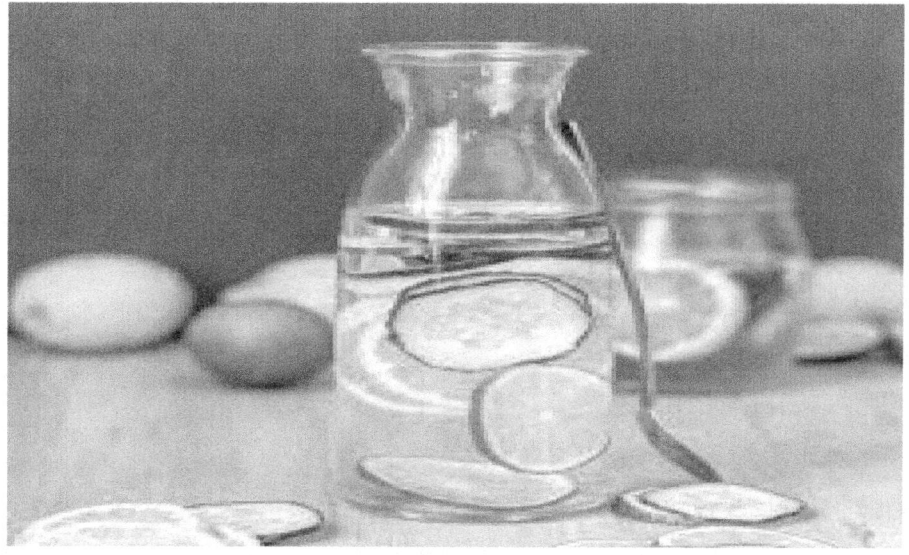

- Total Time: 5 mins

- Prep. Time: 5 mins

- Cooking Time: N/A

- Serving Size: 1 serving

Ingredients:

1. 1 cucumber sliced.

2. 1 lemon sliced.

3. 2 cups water

Instructions:

- In a wide mouth bottle, add the cucumber and lemon slices.

- Slightly warm the water and pour it into the bottle with the slices.

- Refrigerate for 1 or 2 hours and consume throughout the day.

8.6. Ginger Tea

Ginger tea is also antioxidant and good for stomach health. You can consume ginger tea during the fast to enhance fat metabolism.

- Total Time: 5-8 mins

- Prep. Time: 5 mins

- Cooking Time: 5 mins

- Serving Size: 2 servings

Ingredients:

1. 2 ½ cup water

2. 2 tsp ginger juice

3. 1 tsp green tea leaves

Instructions:

- In a saucepan, bring water to boil. Add the green tea leaves and ginger juice.

- Cook for 1 to 2 minutes and take off the flame.

- Pour in cups and enjoy your ginger tea.

8.7. Black Tea

If you are not a coffee drinker but a tea drinker, this recipe is just for you.

- Total Time: 5 mins

- Prep Time: 1 min

- Cooking Time: 4-5 mins

- Serving Size: 2 servings

Ingredients:

1. 1 tsp regular tea
2. 2 ½ cup water

Instructions:

- In a saucepan, bring water to boil.
- Add the tea and let it boil for 2 minutes.
- Now strain the tea and pour it into bowls.

8.8. Bone Broth

Bone broth is rich in vitamins and some fats. Some professionals argue that the presence of fats makes it unsuitable for the fasting window. But some professionals agree that it can be consumed in more severe forms of fasting like 24-hour fasting and Warrior fasting. However, one can decide for themselves if they want to consume it during the fast or not.

- Total Time: 30 mins
- Prep. Time: 10 mins
- Cooking Time: 20 mins
- Serving Size: 1 serving

Ingredients:

1. 3 cups water
2. Few chicken bones without meat
3. ¼ tsp salt
4. ¼ tsp pepper
5. 2 garlic cloves
6. 1 small onion cut in half.

Instructions:

- In a medium saucepan, add together all the ingredients and bring them to a boil.

- Lower the flame and let it simmer for 20 mins.

- Strain the liquid in a cup.

- Your healthy bone broth is ready. Serve while hot.

8.9. Diluted Apple Cider Vinegar

Apple cider vinegar has been known to play an important role in weight loss and boosting fat burn. Some people consume it directly, but it is not recommended because of its strong acidity. You should always dilute to drink it.

- Total Time: 5 mins

- Prep. Time: 5 mins

- Cooking Time: N/A

- Serving Size: 1 serving

Ingredients:

1. 2 tbsp apple cider vinegar

2. 1 glass water

Instructions:

- In a glass full of water, add the apple cider vinegar.

- Mix well and consume it slowly.

- Drinking the whole glass at once can cause acidity.

8.10. Simple Green Tea

Green tea has long been associated with weight loss and stomach health. This is a simple recipe for green tea.

- Total Time: 5 mins

- Prep Time: 2 mins

- Cooking Time: 3-5 mins
- Serving size: 1 serving

Ingredients:

1. 1 tsp dried green tea
2. 1 tsp lemon juice
3. 2 ½ cups water

Instructions:

- Bring water to boil in a saucepan.
- Add the green tea and let it cook for one minute.
- Turn off the flame and pour the tea into cups.
- Add lemon juice to both cups equally, and enjoy your warm tea.

8.11. Raspberry Detox Water

Raspberries are a rich source of vitamins. Having detox water not only ensures hydration but also provides you with essential vitamins as well.

- Total Time: 5 mins
- Prep. Time: 5 mins
- Cooking Time: N/A
- Serving Size: 1 serving

Ingredients:

1. Handful raspberries
2. 2 cups water
3. 1 lemon sliced.

Instructions:

- In a 5ooml wide-mouthed bottle, add the raspberries and lemon slices. Pour water over the fruits.

- Consume throughout the day. You can refill water when the water is finished.

- You can use it for up to 4 hours.

8.12. Mint Detox Water

This is also a simple way you can keep hydrated.

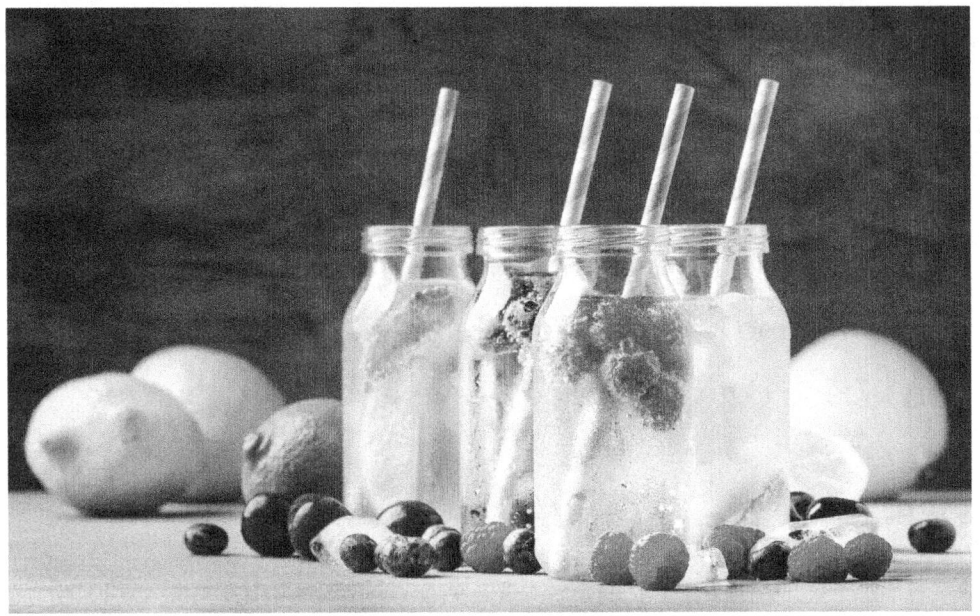

- Total Time: 5 mins

- Prep. Time: 5 mins

- Cooking Time: N/A

- Serving Size: 1 serving

Ingredients:

1. 2 cups water

2. 5-10 mint leaves

3. 1-inch ginger piece

4. 1 lemon sliced.

Instructions:

- Take a 500 ml water bottle with a wide mouth.

- Add the mint, ginger, and lemon slices.

- Pour over the water and chill.

- You can use this water for up to four hours.

8.13. Chamomile Tea

This is a detox drink and gives a soothing effect. You can consume this tea during the fasting window.

- Total Time: 15 mins

- Prep. Time: 2 mins

- Cook Time: 5 mins

- Serving Size: 1 serving

Ingredients:

1. 1 tsp dried chamomile flowers

2. 1 ½ cup water

Instructions:

- In a saucepan, put water and chamomile tea. Bring the water to a boil.

- Boil for 2 minutes and turn off the stove.

- Cover the saucepan and let the tea infuse.

- After 10 minutes, please turn on the flame again and bring it to a boil.

- As soon as tea boils, strain it to your cup and enjoy the tea.

8.14. Blueberry Detox Water

Detox water not only keeps you hydrated but also provides you with essential vitamins.

- Total Time: 5 mins

- Prep. Time: 5 mins

- Cooking Time: N/A

- Serving Size: 1 serving

Ingredients:

1. 10 blueberries
2. 1 lemon sliced.
3. 2 cups water.

Instructions:

- In a 500 ml water bottle, put in the blueberries and the lemon slices.
- Pour over the 2 cups of water.
- Chill in the fridge or put inside some ice cubes.
- This detox water should be consumed within 4 hours.

8.15. Peach Tea

This is a fruit tea. The aroma of this tea gives you a refreshing effect and activates your olfactory chambers. This tea has detoxifying effects as well as positive aromatic effects on the body and mind.

- Total Time: 10 mins
- Prep. Time: 2 mins
- Cooke Time: 8 mins
- Serving Size: 1 serving

Ingredients:

1. 2 tsp dried peach bits
2. 1 lemon
3. 1 ½ cup water

Instructions:

- In a small saucepan, add water and dried peach bits.
- Bring the water to boil ad lower the flame. Let it simmer for 5 to 6 mins.

- Turn off the flame and strain the tea into your cup.

- Squeeze a lemon in the tea to enhance flavors.

- Enjoy your tea.

8.16. Jasmine Tea

- Total Time: 15 mins

- Prep. Time: 2 mins

- Cook Time: 5 mins

- Serving Size: 1 serving

Ingredients:

1. 1 tsp dried jasmine flowers

2. 1 ½ cup water

3. Few mint leaves

Instructions:

- In a saucepan, put water, jasmine tea, and mint leaves. Bring the water to a boil.

- Boil for 2 minutes and turn off the stove.

- Cover the saucepan and let the tea infuse.

- After 10 minutes, please turn on the flame again and bring it to a boil.

- As soon as tea boils, strain it to your cup and enjoy the tea.

8.17. Beef Bone Broth

- Total Time: 30 mins

- Prep. Time: 10 mins

- Cooking Time: 20 mins

- Serving Size: 1 serving

Ingredients:

1. 3 cups water
2. Beef ribs without meat
3. ¼ tsp salt
4. ¼ tsp pepper
5. 2 garlic cloves
6. 1 small onion cut in half.

Instructions:

- In a medium saucepan, add together all the ingredients and bring them to a boil.
- Lower the flame and let it simmer for 20 mins.
- Strain the liquid in a cup.
- Your healthy bone broth is ready. Serve while hot.

8.18. Fish Broth

- Total Time: 30 mins
- Prep. Time: 10 mins
- Cooking Time: 20 mins
- Serving Size: 1 serving

Ingredients:

1. 3 cups water
2. Fishbones without flesh
3. ¼ tsp salt
4. ¼ tsp pepper
5. 2 garlic cloves
6. 1 small onion cut in half.

Instructions:

- In a medium saucepan, add together all the ingredients and bring them to a boil.

- Lower the flame and let it simmer for 20 mins.

- Strain the liquid in a cup.

- Your healthy bone broth is ready. Serve while hot.

8.19. Strawberry Tea

- Total Time: 10 mins

- Prep. Time: 2 mins

- Cooke Time: 8 mins

- Serving Size: 1 serving

Ingredients:

1. 2 tsp dried strawberry bits

2. 1 lemon

3. 1 ½ cup water

Instructions:

- In a small saucepan, add water and dried strawberry bits.

- Bring the water to boil ad lower the flame. Let it simmer for 5 to 6 mins.

- Turn off the flame and strain the tea into your cup.

- Squeeze a lemon in the tea to enhance flavors.

- Enjoy your tea.

8.20. Herbal Tea

- Total Time: 10 mins

- Prep. Time: 2 mins

- Cooke Time: 8 mins

- Serving Size: 2 servings

Ingredients:

1. 5 cup water
2. ¼ tsp clove powder
3. 1 tsp fennel seeds
4. 5 green cardamoms
5. 10 mint leaves
6. ¼ tsp ginger powder

Instructions:

- In a saucepan, bring water to boil.
- Add all the herbs and boil for 2 minutes.
- Turn off the flame and cover the saucepan for 5 minutes so that the herbs can infuse.
- Strain the tea in another saucepan and bring it to boil.
- Serve hot.

8.21. Lemon Grass Tea

- Total Time: 10 mins
- Prep. Time: 2 mins
- Cooke Time: 8 mins
- Serving Size: 1 serving

Ingredients:

1. 2 sticks lemongrass
2. 1 lemon
3. 1 ½ cup water

Instructions:

- In a small saucepan, add water and add lemongrass.

- Bring the water to boil ad lower the flame. Let it simmer for 5 to 6 mins.

- Turn off the flame and strain the tea into your cup.

- Squeeze a lemon in the tea to enhance flavors.

- Enjoy your tea.

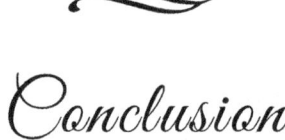

Conclusion

Going on a diet and shift one's focus to a new lifestyle may seem daunting and terrifying. It is human nature to remain in one's comfort zone. But reading this book must have cleared a lot of your doubts about intermittent fasting and how it is the most practical way of life if you are touching your fifties. The best thing about intermittent fasting is that no food groups are off-limits. You can easily schedule your day around your eating routine.

The most practical intermittent fasting routine is the 16:8 structure. It is the most practical and easiest to follow because half of the fast is spent sleeping, making it easier to follow. Another thing about eating is that people tend to eat even when they are hungry; with intermittent fasting, you can drink beverages. In this way, you can keep away from calories as well as keep hydrated.

The recipes in this book are simple and easy to follow and are included in mind the health requirements at age 50. All the recipes are low-calorie, and most of them incorporate healthy ingredients. The smoothies included in the drinks chapter are high in calcium content which is an essential requirement for ladies.

This book must have motivated you to develop this new lifestyle with numerous health benefits.

COOKING CONVERSION CHART

Measurement

CUP	ONCES	MILLILITERS	TABLESPOONS
8 cup	64 oz	1895 ml	128
6 cup	48 oz	1420 ml	96
5 cup	40 oz	1180 ml	80
4 cup	32 oz	960 ml	64
2 cup	16 oz	480 ml	32
1 cup	8 oz	240 ml	16
3/4 cup	6 oz	177 ml	12
2/3 cup	5 oz	158 ml	11
1/2 cup	4 oz	118 ml	8
3/8 cup	3 oz	90 ml	6
1/3 cup	2.5 oz	79 ml	5.5
1/4 cup	2 oz	59 ml	4
1/8 cup	1 oz	30 ml	3
1/16 cup	1/2 oz	15 ml	1

Temperature

FAHRENHEIT	CELSIUS
100 °F	37 °C
150 °F	65 °C
200 °F	93 °C
250 °F	121 °C
300 °F	150 °C
325 °F	160 °C
350 °F	180 °C
375 °F	190 °C
400 °F	200 °C
425 °F	220 °C
450 °F	230 °C
500 °F	260 °C
525 °F	274 °C
550 °F	288 °C

Weight

IMPERIAL	METRIC
1/2 oz	15 g
1 oz	29 g
2 oz	57 g
3 oz	85 g
4 oz	113 g
5 oz	141 g
6 oz	170 g
8 oz	227 g
10 oz	283 g
12 oz	340 g
13 oz	369 g
14 oz	397 g
15 oz	425 g
1 lb	453 g

Made in the USA
Monee, IL
11 May 2021